A New Look at Vegetarianism:

It's Positive Effects on Health and Disease Control

Dr. Sukhraj S. Dhillon, Ph. D.

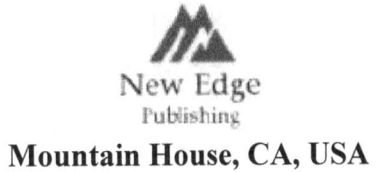

New Edge
Publishing

Mountain House, CA, USA

Other Titles and their ISBNs under Self-help and Spiritual Series:
"The Power of Breathing" (ISBN: 978-1466371545)
"A Simple Solution to America's Weight Problem" (ISBN: 978-1466377127)
"Art of Stress-Free Living:" (ISBN: 978-1481850131)
"Forever Young" (ISBN: 978-1466392069)
"A New Look at Vegetarianism:" (ISBN: 978-1482560916)
"Health, Happiness & Longevity:" (ISBN: 0870405276)
"Soul and Reincarnation" (ISBN: 978-1466395930)
"Science, Religion & Spirituality" (ISBN: 978-1482033236)
"In Search of God" (ISBN: 978-1466398498)
"A Treasure of Great Spiritual Stories" (ISBN: 978-1466394773)
"Industrial Leaks and Air Pollution:" (ISBN: 9997691547)
"Cigarette Smoking:" (ISBN: 9997691547)

Revised Edition Printed: 2013
ISBN-13: 978-1482560916
ISBN-10: 1482560917

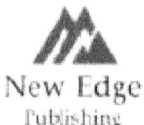

New Edge
Publishing
www.newedgepublishing.com
Printed in U.S.A.

© Dr. Sukhraj S. Dhillon, Ph.D.
First Published 1993 by: Oakwood Pub Co./P P I Publishing
ISBN 1575150298
Printed in the USA
Revised "2004, 2007, 2013"

CONTENTS

INTRODUCTION

When we look at eating patterns today, we can see diets that have been proven to work over centuries of experience, and diets which have been deliberately constructed over the past few years, based on fad, fancy, and many times experimental evidence. In nutrition, as in other areas of science, we find many different views. The reason, most often, is that particular information gained through scientific studies does not and perhaps cannot, take into consideration all possible complications that may set in due to the inherently complex nature of biological systems. For example, at one time carbohydrates were recommended to help us burn fat. Now again carbohydrates are labeled to make us fat in Atkinson's diet. The high protein diet recommendations took us away from fruits and vegetables which, along with fiber, are actually necessary to maintain good health and proper weight.

The recent suggestions to cut down on processed foods with high salt and sugar content and increased intake of fresh fruits and vegetables to achieve and maintain proper weight and good health, are not really new. On examining common eating practices in earlier societies we find that these had always been a part of their diet. Moreover, humans have biologically evolved with a diet which includes wholesome foods in their natural state, primarily of plant origin; these are just the kind of foods with fruits and vegetables that are associated with good health by recent findings.

The consumption of excessive meat and processed foods leads to an unbalanced diet, since they contain a great excess of protein, yet are almost completely lacking in carbohydrates, fiber, calcium, and health-promoting vitamins, originally derived from the plant kingdom. However, these missing ingredients, essential parts of good nutrition, can be provided by fresh vegetables, fruits, grains, and dairy products. A wholesome vegetarian diet, in fact, can supply all of the nutrition necessary for the human body. Perhaps it is not surprising that vegetarians have enjoyed good health for centuries. There are several examples of long-lived people-the Hunzans of Pakistan, the Abkhasians of the Soviet Union, and the

Vilcabambams of Ecuador-whose diets contain little animal foods. While many factors, including high levels of exercise and low levels of stress, undoubtedly contribute to the longevity of these people, their wholesome vegetarian diet is likely to be a very significant factor. The "secret" of their natural diet is now supported by the medical and scientific world that has recently realized, as stated above, the importance of fresh fruits and vegetables, and the need for moderation in protein consumption to maintain good health.

The influence of wholesome foods on our health goes even further. For instance, while methods of weight control range from fad diets to behavior modification, the final answer to getting thin and staying thin seems to lie in adopting a diet of wholesome foods. Widespread adoption of this approach could save the United States alone over 10 billion dollars, the sum spent annually on weight reduction efforts (According to data published by G.A. Bray. *Recent Advances in Obesity Research, II.* Newman Publishing, London. p. 248-265). Vast as it is, the 10 billion dollar figure does not even include the medical costs resulting from obesity related diseases.

In view of rising medical care costs, Ex-U.S. Secretary of Health and Human Resources Richard Schweicker has noted that prevention and more rational approaches to diseases and aging are mandatory. Approximately 100,000 coronary by-passes are performed yearly at an average cost of $50,000 each ($5 billion) and 1,000 people in the U.S. alone die every day of cancer. Some of the heart operations can be avoided by putting patients on proper diet and exercise programs, as is already being realized by some of the heart specialists in the United States. Furthermore, the carotenoids and retinoids provided by certain vegetables (orange and yellow plant chemicals related to vitamin A) appear to offer important cancer prevention properties during the twenty-to-thirty-year lag phase in the development of human cancer, even after exposure has occurred. Japanese epidemiologists have shown that cigarette smokers who eat green and yellow vegetables have 30% less cancer, compared to appropriately matched controls who do not eat these retinoid-and carotenoid-containing vegetables. A prudent diet that is low in fats and high in fresh fruits and vegetables is desirable, as is control over disease-provoking habits such as smoking, alcoholism and obesity.

A natural diet with plenty of vegetables and fruits can give sick people a new lease on life and save others from common diseases such as colon cancer and heart trouble. These foods can improve the vigor and vitality of those already in good health and contribute to their overall efficiency. We can go further and use these foods in prolonging life. In practicing the eating habits put forward in the pages of this guide, the reader, it is hoped, will be able to enjoy a long disease-free life, full of health and vigor.

Chapter 1

VEGETARIANISM AND WHY CONSIDER IT

The most popular types of vegetarian diets are fruits and vegetables supplemented with dairy foods (and sometimes eggs and even fish). However, since vegetarian diets vary and are identified with certain standard terms, it is appropriate to define some of these here. The vegetarians who eat fruits and vegetables only are called VEGANS. The others who eat fruits, vegetables and dairy products are called LACTOVEGETARIANS, and those who eat eggs in addition to lactovegetarian foods are called LACTO-OVOVEGETARIANS. The healthy, vegetarian diet emphasized in this guide is probably close to that of lactovegetarians if they consume wholesome, unprocessed, unpreserved foods. For example, brown rice, not white; whole wheat, not refined flour; fresh, not canned vegetables; and fruits, not fruit juices. Eaten raw or cooked, these foods are low in fats, cholesterol, protein, and highly refined carbohydrates such as sugars. They are high in mostly unrefined carbohydrates such as starches. These foods are not only safe and healthy, but are ideal for maintaining a proper weight level-without any restrictions on food quantity.

Many Americans are used to convenience foods, which may make the first step towards healthful vegetarian foods seem difficult. However, once that step is taken, and the food is tried and the rewards are understood, then the chances of adopting a vegetarian diet are good. The process can be a gradual one, with adoption of various ingredients of the diet taking place at whatever pace is comfortable.

Wholesome plant foods are actually better suited to our bodies than are foods made popular by recent trends in eating. These natural foods are the basic foods which were available while our physiology evolved to its present complexity; these foods are in harmony with our digestive and metabolic machinery evolved over thousands of years.

Why Adopt A Vegetarian Diet?

Vegetarian foods provide an effective method of reducing the dangers of an over-rich diet; nutritionally, you have nothing to lose. Recognition of vegetarianism as a part of health and longevity is now spreading. The number of voluntary vegetarians in Europe and the USA is estimated at several million. Some are motivated by aesthetic or moral ideas; they deplore the killing of animals and some of the methods of raising them for food. Many become vegetarians for hygienic reasons, spurning meat as a cause of digestive problems and disease, and a source of unhealthy chemicals and infectious organisms. Others simply believe that a vegetarian diet is more healthy. The unprocessed vegetarian foods are low in fat and cholesterol but are high in starchy carbohydrates and fiber, and natural vitamins and minerals. The vegetable proteins can be as satisfying as meat protein. Proper combinations of vegetarian foods for good quality protein are explained in chapter 2.

For centuries the hardiest, most long-lived people in the world have thrived on these foods. President Thomas Jefferson, who lived to be eighty-three, believed his longevity was due to his vegetarian menus. He wrote, "I have lived temperately, eating little animal food, and not as an aliment, so much as a condiment for the vegetables which constitute my principal diet." Among other famous vegetarians were George Bernard Shaw, Leonardo da Vinci, Ralph Waldo Emerson, Henry David Thoreau, Benjamin Franklin, Mahatma Gandhi, Albert Schweitzer, Gloria Swanson, and Michael Jackson.

My grand-mother who lived to be over 90 years of age never consumed meat, fish or eggs. Her diet was wholesome grains, vegetables, some fruits and dairy products. Even among dairy her main drink was butter milk. She never went to a doctor or dentist. She didn't fall sick at the time of death. She was found expired next morning. She had most of her natural teeth at the time of death. I am sure, genetics played a role but her eating habits cannot be ignored.

Vegetarian foods are not only healthy but are economical, so that even the poorest can afford them. Meat, on the other hand, is an expensive and inefficient nutrient. It is more efficient to use land for growing food for humans directly than for feeding animals which then are used as food. Table 1.1 shows how many people, for the same period, could be supported by 10 acres of land in terms of vegetarian proteins compared with meat proteins. A 1,000 lb. steer eats 5,250 lbs. of plant food in its lifetime. Its carcass weighs only 560 lb. and from this the consumer will be able to buy only 280 lbs. of prime cuts of its meat, quite a significant reduction in the amount of available food.

In view of the world-wide population explosion, our protein must come more and more from non-meat sources. Highly populated countries, such as China and India, for centuries have used more vegetable protein than animal protein. Less populated countries are now beginning to face the same problem. In the future, vegetable protein foods, such as soybean products, are likely to become more important in our diet because they are cheaper to produce than animal protein (see Table 1.1). The ever increasing demand for protein can never be solved through meat, because the world's resources are too limited to squander on the uneconomical conversion of plant to animal to human protein. Increasingly, people all over the world will have to rely on vegetable proteins. If we all increased the use of vegetable proteins, food would be cheaper and more abundant.

Table 1.1. The economics of vegetarianism. The number of people fed by 10 acres of land in terms of vegetarian proteins compared with meat proteins.

Source of Protein	No. of People Fed per 10 Acres
Soybean	61
Wheat	24
Corn	10
Meat	2

Even if we are not concerned about the world food problem, dealing every day with the steadily rising cost of food, especially of meat and fish, is a good enough reason to learn about utilization of plant proteins. Table 1.2 shows the relative cost of 54 grams of protein (the daily recommended dietary allowance of protein for a 150-pound adult). These figures are based on January, 1980 prices by the U.S. Department of Agriculture and Labor. These will vary from time to time but should give a sense of the relative cost of our protein needs. Ounce for ounce, the protein in bologna costs four times as much as the protein in peanut butter. The protein in bacon is about five times, in beef about seven times and in lamb chops about nine times as expensive as the same amount of protein from kidney beans.

Table 1.2. The relative cost of 54 grams of protein from plant and animal sources, the daily recommended dietary allowance of protein for a 150-pound adult.

Food	Amount	Cost (January 1980)
Dried beans, cooked	3 2/5 cup	$0.38
Peanut butter	13 1/2 Tbsp.	0.54
Eggs	11 large	0.62
Chicken, whole	7/10 small broiler	0.73
Tuna, canned	71/2 ounces	1.08
Frankfurters	8 medium	1.65
Sardines, canned	10 ounces	1.73
Bacon, sliced	21 1/2 ounces	1.92
Bologna	16 ounces	2.16
Beef sirloin, w/ bone	12 ounces	2.21
Veal cutlets	9 1/2 ounces	2.81
Porterhouse steak, with bone	15 ounces	3.16
Lamb chops, loin	13 1/2 ounces	3.48

SOURCE: U.S. Department of Agriculture and Labor.

Vegetarian foods provide an additional advantage of "eating low on the food chain." The higher on the food chain you eat, the greater your chances of accumulating large amounts of toxic materials present in tiny amounts in foods at the bottom of the chain. Meat protein, in fact, is called second-hand protein because the animal eats the vegetation, a primary source of protein, to build up its own protein which is then utilized by the meat eater who eats the animal. The carnivorous animal protein is thus third hand and is often toxic to consume, and this is the reason that the meat people eat usually comes from vegetarian animals (for example, grain fed beef). Although fish appears to be an exception, health conscious people prefer small fish such as sardines, which are lower on the food chain, to bigger fish such as tuna. The reason is that big fish eat smaller fish, each with some pollutants or other toxins stored in its body, and therefore small fish at the lower end of the food chain are less likely to contain any pollutants or other toxic substances. This is, in fact, what has happened to birds of prey like falcons, ospreys, and eagles who eat big fish. These birds at the top of the food chain end up taking in such a large amount of pesticides such as DDT (banned now in many countries but replaced with other pesticides) that their reproductive ability is severely damaged. The advantages of eating at the lower end of the food chains has been substantiated by the data published in *Pesticides Monitoring Journal;* the plant foods at the lower end of the food chain contain less pesticide residues than foods of animal origin. Vegetarians go right to the beginning of the food chain and from nuts, seeds, beans, grains, and vegetables, they get protein first-hand from nature.

One could cite numerous reasons for eating vegetarian foods, but the one we would emphasize in this guide is simply that vegetarian food is good for you to enjoy the best of health. I would quote the common responses of many vegetarian people who refer to their personal experience rather than any nutritional aspects: (1) although the main requirement for being a vegetarian is not eating meat, vegetarianism is more like an entire relationship with the world-a sensitive vibration; it is a spiritual position that we have arrived at-as our place here on earth, (2) there is something violent about meat-eating; you are constantly slaughtering animals for your gastronomic pleasure, (3) there is something nice and clean about eating grains; they are good for your body, (4) meat-eaters tend to "break" because they are not as adaptable; meat-eating leaves one feeling very heavy and sluggish; it also makes people more aggressive, (5) vegetarians have high levels of endurance and can work for longer hours.

Natural Human Diet according to Biological and Evolutionary Evidence

The foods and influences to which a species is biologically adapted are those deemed "natural" to its disposition as derived by the sum total of their biological heritage from millions of years of evolution. Cumulative adaptations in each species over eons of time determines their natural dietary needs. For instance: The koala bear of Australia is adapted to eating a variety of gum leaves. The giraffe's long neck allows it to feed on the foliage of trees. The lion's fangs and claws allow it to kill and render animals for food. The eagle's keen eyesight and powerful claws make it a formidable predator of ground rodents and small game. Carnivores have become adapted to eating other animals. Non-carnivorous animals have adapted to eating vegetable matter as food. Dietary adaptations more than anything else determine the features and characteristics of all creatures.

Animal species classified on the basis of their natural biologically evolved diets. {Dietary terms associated with vegetarianism}

Term	Primary Food	Animal Species
Herbivores	Equipped to handle raw leaf/grass	grazers- cattle, rabbits, horses, sheep, etc.
Granivores	raw grains of various grasses	primarily birds
Frugivores	thrive mostly on raw fruits, succulent fruit-like vegetables, roots, shoots, nuts and seeds	apes, gorillas, chimpanzees, monkeys, orangutans etc.
Carnivores	eat raw meat	cats, lions, tigers, wolves, etc.
Insectivores	thrive on insects	ant-eaters, amphibians, other insect eaters
Omnivores	every food from plant or animal	hogs, brown bears, raccoons, etc.

Humans Are Not an Exception

It is a basic premise of Natural Hygiene that humans, like all other creatures in nature are provided with all the materials and conditions required to maintain health. Species throughout nature intuitively restrict themselves to a limited variety of foods to which they are specifically adapted. We must conclude that humans are also intended to partake only of those foods to which we are physiologically adapted in order to live healthfully. Humans should be studied as a member of the whole biological community, and compared anatomically and physiologically with other species to ascertain our true dietary requirements. When considering the character of human anatomy and physiology relative to our natural diet we must do so within the context of nature, rather than in the artificial environment of modern life. In this way, we consider our natural foods as those that are consonant with our physiological faculties, rather than those that we have "acquired a taste for".

Determining Our Natural Diet is Not a Matter of Belief.

Tradition and popularity are the poorest ways to determine a proper diet. Recent changes in our external environment do not alter our biological adaptations, our internal makeup, or our natural needs in order to establish optimum well-being. Biological adaptations have been spurred on by stress over eons of time and by the need to adapt. They are slow to develop requiring extremely long periods of time to evolve. Our highly industrialized environment involves more social adaptations or accommodations, and not physical or anatomical changes. By living according to our natural adaptations we can actually withstand the stress of modern life far better than if we transgress our biological needs.

The only authority we should rely on when it comes to determining what foods are best to eat is the human body. It is anatomy and physiology that decrees whether food is "acceptable" or "harmful". Determining our natural diet is not a matter of belief: its basis lies in scientific fact regarding our biological, biochemical, anatomical, and physiological features.

The first question in forming a scientific opinion about our natural diet is: What is our natural food? Are we true carnivores who secure their nutrient needs not only from raw flesh, but also from raw blood, bones etc, as tigers and wolves? Are we true herbivores (grazers) who thrive on lettuce, grasses, raw grains, celery, etc., as do horses, cows and sheep? Are we granivores like birds who thrive mostly on raw seeds of grasses and grains? Are we natural omnivores who thrive in health regardless of the foodstuffs consumed? Or are we frugivores who can thrive on a diet of raw fresh bananas, grapes, apples, oranges, or melons meal after meal?

The human digestive system and physiology determines our optimum diet. By understanding the physiological processes that accompany food digestion and absorption, proper dietary habits can be scientifically determined.

Teeth Comparison

Most "nutritionists" assert that we have definite carnivorous leanings, and some have even termed our incisor teeth "fangs" in defense of their erroneous position that humans are natural meat-eaters! If you look at the various species in the animal kingdom, each is equipped with teeth that are ideally suited to masticate a particular type of food. Herbivores (like the cow) have 24 molars, eight jagged incisors in the lower jaw and a horny palate in the upper jaw. Their jaws move vertically, laterally, forward, and backward, enabling the herbivore to tear and grind coarse grasses. Omnivores (like the hog) have tusk-like canines allowing them to dig up roots. Frugivores (like the chimpanzee) have 32 teeth: sixteen in each jaw including four incisors, two cuspids, four bicuspids, and six molars. The cuspids are adapted for cracking nuts, and the uniform articulation of the teeth enables the frugivore to mash and grind fruits. On the contrary, carnivores (like the cat family) have markedly developed canines that are long, sharp, cylindrical, pointed, and set apart from the other teeth. Fangs and sharp pointed teeth that penetrate and kill, that rip and tear flesh, are a feature of all true carnivores (except certain birds). The powerful jaws of the carnivore move only vertically, and are ideal for ripping and tearing flesh that is swallowed virtually whole and then acted upon by extremely potent gastric juices. **Human teeth are not designed for tearing flesh as in the lion, wolf or dog, but rather compare closely with other fruit-eating animals. Human teeth correspond almost identically to the chimpanzees and other frugivores.** The complete absence of spaces between human teeth characterizes us as the archetype frugivore. The "canine" teeth of humans are short, stout, and slightly triangular. They are less pronounced and developed than the orangutan's, who rarely kills and eats raw flesh in its natural environment. Human canines in no way resemble the long, round, slender canines of the true carnivore. Human teeth are not curved or sharp like the wolves or tigers, nor are they wide and flat like the grass and grain-eating species. Human teeth are actually like the fruit-eating monkeys, and the human mouth is best suited for eating succulent fruits and vegetables. It would be extremely difficult, if not impossible, for humans to eat raw flesh without the aid of fork and knife. To term our incisor teeth "fangs" or even to liken them as such is outrageous.

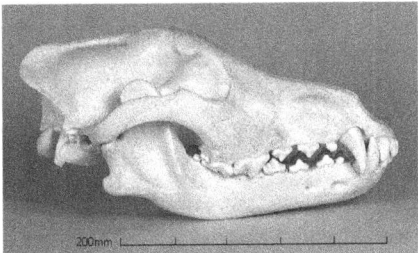
Wolf

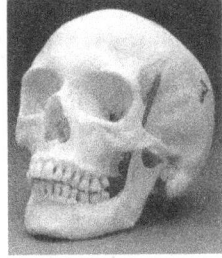
Human

Comparative Anatomy
Natural carnivores have the inherent anatomical equipment provided as their birthright with which to apprehend, capture, kill, and rend their quarry. Dogs have powerful jaws that inflict fatal wounds to their prey. Humans however, have no sharp claws for tearing; no sharply pointed fangs for slashing; nor are our eyes or olfactory senses well developed for hunting. Nor is the human body designed to run fast enough to capture prey. Humans cannot grab animals in their mouth as do dogs, coyotes, wolves, jackals, lions, tigers, or cats. We instead inflict more damage with our hands and brute strength. Humans do however, have marvelous fingers, thumbs, and

limbs for reaching, climbing and grabbing. Our natural food gathering capacity is very similar to the chimpanzees. Fruitarians of the primate order also have revolving joints in their shoulder, wrist, and elbow joints that allow for free movement in all directions. Frugivores have soft pliable, sensitive hands and fingers with opposable thumbs and flat nails that are perfect for grasping and gathering fruit.

Regarding the extremities of the other species, herbivores possess hooves allowing them to walk easily about grassy plains, and carnivores possess sharp claws allowing them to violently attack their prey. Tree-dwellers and fruit-gatherers also have stereoscopic binocular vision that makes vision precise enough to ascertain the position of tree limbs and objects.

Another anatomical comparison among species in the animal kingdom involves the structure of the skin. All vegetarian animals have abundant sweat glands. In carnivores, their sweat glands are atrophied and inactive. They are exempt from profuse sweating in order to prevent a large fluid loss that would cause concentrated precipitation of nitrogenous wastes (from flesh-eating). This explains why mcat-eaters suffer in hot weather while vegetarians remain relatively comfortable.

Comparative Digestive Physiology
Among the various species throughout nature, the length of their particular alimentary canals also differs greatly in relation to their natural food. The gut of the carnivore is 3-6 times the length of their body. They require a short, smooth, fast-acting gut since their natural flesh diet becomes quite toxic and cannot be retained within the intestine for long without poisonous putrefaction taking place. The gut of the herbivore is sacculated for greater surface area, and is 30 times the length of their body. Its herb and grass diet is coarse and fibrous, requiring longer digestion to break down cellulose. The length of the omnivore's alimentary canal is generally 6 times its body trunk size. The gut of the frugivore (like humans) is also sacculated and is 12 times the length of its body. The human digestive tract is about four times as long as the carnivores. The

intestine of the carnivore is short and smooth in order to dissolve food rapidly and pass it quickly out of the system prior to the flesh putrefying. The human digestive tract is corrugated for the specific purpose of retaining food as long as possible until all nutriment has been extracted, which is the worst possible condition for the digestion and processing of flesh foods. Meat moves quickly through the carnivore's digestive tract and is quickly expelled. The human lengthy intestine cannot handle low-fiber foods including meat and dairy very quickly at all. As a consequence, animal foods decrease the motility of the human intestine and putrefaction almost invariably occurs (as evidenced by foul smelling stools and flatulence), resulting in the release of many poisonous by-products as the low-fiber food passes through, ever so slowly. In humans, eventual constipation may develop on a meat-centered diet. Colon cancer is also common, both of which are rare or non-existent on a high-fiber diet centered around raw fruits and vegetables.

Stomach, Kidney and Liver!
Stomach form and size among various species also vary markedly. In the carnivore the stomach is a small, round sack designed to dissolve flesh quickly and then pass it on for removal. In plant eaters (particularly ruminants) stomachs are complicated adjoining sacks with ring-like convolutions. The frugivore stomach (including humans) is oblong and is characterized by folds called rugae which serve to retain food for relatively long periods.

Organ sizes of various species also markedly vary. The liver and kidneys in the carnivore are much larger than in vegetarian animals. A lions kidney is twice the size of a bulls, and not much smaller than the elephants. This allows the lion to handle large amounts of protein and nitrogenous waste products contained in its natural flesh diet. The carnivores huge liver secretes larger amounts of bile into the small intestine than does the herbivores liver. There is a direct relation between the quantity of meat eaten and the amount of bile secreted. Meat-eating therefore, places a strain on the small liver of humans which impairs the organ's function over a long period of time.

When you place humans on a diet for which they are NOT naturally adapted, this places unnatural stress on the organs of elimination. Humans have never adapted to the carnivorous diet that is high in animal products. The human liver is smaller than the carnivores and as a result, we cannot detoxify the poisonous products inherent within animal foods such as uric acid (discussed below). Our kidneys are also smaller and become diseased from overwork caused by a diet high in animal protein.

Comparative Digestive Enzymes

The hydrochloric acid concentrations of various species are an additional determinant of their natural diet. A carnivores gastric juice is highly acidic, serving to prevent putrefaction while flesh undergoes digestion. Plant-eaters however, secrete a much less concentrated and less abundant quantity of hydrochloric acid that does not curtail the bacterial decomposition of flesh: a process that begins at the animals moment of death. Flesh is digested in an acid medium within the stomach. Humans secrete a very weak concentration of hydrochloric acid relative to the carnivore, and little of the protein-splitting enzyme pepsinogen. Carnivorous animals have concentrations of these flesh-digesting secretions 1100% greater than do humans. Lions can rip off and swallow your hand whole and quite readily digest it.

Uric Acid: Toxic Component of Meat to Humans

About 5% of the flesh volume of all animals consists of waste material called uric acid that is normally eliminated by the kidneys. Uric acid is a poison to humans because it is toxic and non-metabolizable. Nearly 100% of Americans suffer some form of osteoporosis which is due in large part, to the acidic end-products of meat (and grain) eating. All carnivorous animals however, secrete the enzyme uricase that breaks down uric acid so it can be readily eliminated. Humans do not generate this enzyme. Instead, we ABSORB uric acid when meat is eaten. As a result, calcium-urate crystals form and concentrate in joints, feet, and in the lower back. These deposits lead to arthritis, gout, rheumatism, bursitis, and lower back pain. Humans are physiologically unsuited to utilizing meat as food. Natural carnivores swallow hunks of carrion almost unchewed, and the flesh is digested in the stomach with ease and facility. If humans were to do the same, we would digest very little of it before putrefaction set in and illness ensued. For humans, meat is a pathogenic and nutritionally deficient food.

Saliva pH Varies Widely Among Species

The saliva pH of various species is another determinant of their natural diet. In carnivores, their saliva glands are small and secrete an acidic saliva having little or no effect on starch, which makes sense since flesh is virtually starch-free. Omnivores (like pigs) have tremendous salivary glands that secrete copious quantities of starch-splitting enzymes. Humans only have one starch-splitting enzyme, versus a multitude of them in omnivores and other natural starch-eating animals. Our ptyalin is very limited. This rules us out as being true granivores (starch-eaters) which includes grains and cereals. Frugivores have salivary glands that secrete alkaline saliva, containing only moderate amounts of ptyalin, which initiates starch digestion. This tells us that humans and other frugivores can easily digest the small amount of starch contained in fresh fruits, nuts, and leafy greens, and that humans are not intended to subsist on a diet of highly starchy grain foods as many currently do. (Diabetes mellitus is largely the result of consuming large amounts of refined sugars and starches. Even eating predominantly of whole grains and natural legumes as dietary staples can be injurious because of the need for excessive starch digestion).

Science Verifies That Human Ancestors Were Frugivores

Dr. Alan Walker, an anthropologist of John Hopkins University in Maryland, has done research showing that early humans were once exclusively fruit eaters. By careful examination of fossil teeth and fossilized human remains with electron microscopes and other sophisticated tools, Dr. Walker and his colleagues are absolutely certain that early humans until relatively recently, were total fruitarians. Source: New York Time, May 15, 1979.

"The natural food of man, judging from his structure, appears to consist principally of the fruits, roots, and other succulent parts of vegetables. His hands afford every facility for gathering them; his

short but moderately strong jaws on the other hand, and his canines being equal only in length to the other teeth, together with his tuberculated molars on the other, would scarcely permit him either to masticate herbage, or to devour flesh, were these condiments not previously prepared by cooking."
-- **Georges Cuvier (1769-1832), Regne Animal, Vol 1, p73**

In conclusion, **our natural diet should consist primarily of fruits, nuts, and green vegetables. We can be called frugivores because many "vegetables" are botanically considered fruits.**

Frugivores are physiologically equipped to obtain energy primarily from the natural sugar in fruits. Humans are bestowed with a kind of "natural sweet tooth" to guide us in the selection of foods that meet our biological disposition and our caloric needs: namely, sweet juicy fruits. Our anatomy is such that we are capable of picking fruits, masticate, digest, and appropriate them with ease and efficiency. Fruits contain all the nutrients we need: vitamins, minerals, proteins (in the form of amino acids), fats, and carbohydrates. All seed-bearing foods are botanically defined as "fruit". This includes avocado, sweet pepper, cucumber, tomato, eggplant, even nuts and seeds.

In Botany fruit is mature ovary, and is made of two parts: the pericarp or edible flesh, and the seed portion itself from fertilized ovules.

To enjoy an energetic, youthful, disease-free life, eat a varied diet predominantly of foods you are biologically adapted to: raw fresh fruits, vegetables, nuts, seeds, sprouted grains, and perhaps occasional legumes and tubers. For more on definition and kinds of vegetables, and health tips including yoga, breathing, aging theories, see Dhillon, S.S. *"Health, Happiness & Longevity: Eastern and Western Approach"* (ISBN: 0870405276). Harper & Row, USA/Japan Publications, Inc., Tokyo, Japan [1983]
http://www.amazon.com/s/ref=br_ss_hs/002-9285375-1842417?platform=gurupa&url=index%3Dblended&keywords=sukhraj+dhillon&Go.x=12&Go.y=9

What Does Biological and Evolutionary Evidence Tell Us About Being Vegetarians or Meat Eaters?

Here's further confirmation that biological and evolutionary evidence put us more towards being vegetarians. Although human beings are considered as **omnivores** who can eat both plant and animal food, our anatomical equipment leans heavily towards a vegetarian diet.

Our teeth are evolved to deal with tubers and seeds, not flesh. Our front teeth are large and sharp, good for biting; our canines are small-almost vestigial compared to a tiger's; our molars are flattened; and our jaws are mobile for grinding food into the small bits we are able to swallow. In contrast, carnivores have long, strong, pointed canine teeth; their upper premolars and lower molars are also large and better designed for cutting than grinding, these slice through flesh like a pair of shears; their jaw moves very little from side to side, limiting their ability to grind food. Dr. Alan Walker of Johns Hopkins University conducted microscopic analyses of the wear patterns on the teeth of our human like ancestors, which indicate that we have evolved from fruit eaters, not flesh eaters. The fossil teeth of these early hominids contain none of the scratch marks found on the teeth of animals that gnaw on bones and flesh.

As for the digestive tract, here, too, we are more like the herbivores. Carnivores have a comparatively short, smooth intestinal tract, only about three times the length of their bodies. Since they eat raw meat that decomposes rapidly, they must digest it fast and get rid of the wastes before toxins accumulate. The human intestines are long (twelve times as long as the torso) and highly convoluted, allowing us to digest substances that take a long time to be broken down and absorbed. Plant foods, with their large amounts of fiber, are just such substances. But whether plant or animal, food takes its time passing through the human digestive system. This leaves animal waste in the body for far longer than it remains in carnivores, and as discussed later in chapter 4, this fact may be related to the high rates of cancer of the colon and rectum among people who eat a lot of meat.

Early humans required meat at times for survival, but analyses of fossilized human fecal matter shows that they subsisted mainly on vegetation fruits, nuts, tubers, berries, and grains. The invention of agriculture, the cultivation of crops for food, further assured a steady supply of edible plants for our ancestors. But it was a long time before animals were domesticated and raised for food, and even then, they were infrequently consumed. More likely they served as suppliers of such renewable foods as milk and eggs. In conclusion, we are biologically constructed as vegetarians, not as consumers of vast quantities of meat.

Chapter 2

NUTRITIONAL CONSIDERATION OF A VEGETARIAN DIET

Before considering the nutritional values of a vegetarian diet, it is appropriate to give a brief review of nutrients and their role in our diet. Nutrients by definition are the life-sustaining constituents in food and nutrition is the process by which living organisms receive and utilize food. The 50 or so known nutrients include proteins (amino acids), carbohydrates (sugar and starches), fats (fatty acids), minerals, vitamins, and water (not a nutrient in a calorie-producing sense). Each of these is needed for proper functioning of the body. They are all essential for the building, upkeep, and repair of body tissues as well as for the efficient functioning of the body. Nutrients are also essential to provide energy for work and play, to move, to breathe, to keep the heart beating, just to be alive, and for supporting growth in children and youth. Although the nutrients are widely distributed in our foods, no single food, not even milk, meat or eggs, contains all the nutrients. Table 2.1 lists the major classes of nutrients, and their main functions and food sources. This basic knowledge about nutrients and their role in our diet is helpful to understand and evaluate vegetarian diets.

The Vegetarian diets have been looked at with skepticism, primarily due to overemphasis on high-protein consumption by meat oriented food writers of the western world. Vegetarians in Europe and America are like left-handed people in a right-handed world. Almost all vegetarians and those thinking of becoming one, are most concerned about getting an adequate supply of protein. If you are on a reasonably well-balanced diet, you need have no fear of getting inadequate protein. A vegetarian diet can be nutritionally sound for all age groups, differing from a non-vegetarian diet only in the sort of foods supplying the essential nutrients. Although the body must get a sufficient supply of these life-sustaining chemicals, their source, whether from meat or non-meat foods, does not matter at all.

Table 2.1. The major classes of nutrients, their main functions and food sources.

Nutrient	% Body Weight	Functions	Main food sources
Proteins	18	Build, repair tissue, regulate body processes, supply energy, fight infection.	Meat, fish, poultry, dried beans, peas, seeds, nuts, cheese, eggs, cereal grains.
Carbohydrates	0.7	Supply energy, spare protein, aid in burning of fat, provide fiber.	Grains, fruits, vegetables, milk.
Fats	15	Provide the essential fatty acid (linoleic acid), promotes absorption of fat-soluble vitamins (A,D,E,K), supply energy.	Fats and oils, nuts, meat, fish, poultry, dairy products, some seeds.
Minerals	3	Regulate body processes, maintain body tissues.	All foods except sugar, alcohol and refined fats and oils.
Vitamins	0.04	Regulate body processes, maintain body tissues and functions.	All foods except sugar, alcohol and refined fats and oils.

Water	63	Transport nutrients, regulates body temperature, participates in chemical reactions, removes waste material.	Water, beverages, and almost all foods have some water.

The statistical data on athletic records indicates that players on vegetarian diets performed as well or even better than those on high-meat diets. Back in 1904, vegetarian and non-vegetarian students were compared as to how many times they could squeeze a grip meter in quick succession. The vegetarians scored an average of 69 times; the non-vegetarians averaged 38. More recently, nine Swedish athletes tested for endurance on a stationary bicycle lasted nearly three times longer after a three-day diet high in vegetables and grains but low in protein than they did after three days of a high-meat diet. If you are still not convinced, note the achievements of vegetarian athletes recounted by Vic Sussman in his book, A *Vegetarian Alternative*. Paava Nurmi, a Finn, trained on a vegetarian diet, and set twenty world running records between 1920 and 1932. Bill Pickering, a British vegetarian, swam the English Channel in 1956 in record-breaking time. Murray Rose, an Australian who had been a vegetarian since the age of 2, at age 17 became the youngest Olympic triple gold medal winner for swimming events in 1956. The point is that you can stay healthy and strong on vegetarian diets.

The following pages provide guidelines for proper food combinations to ensure a nutritional balance of vegetarian foods.

Balancing for Protein Quality

The quality of mixed cereal and legume proteins matches that of non-vegetarian diets, provided proper combination of foods and adequate quantities are consumed. For example, if you depend entirely on white rice for your protein, you would most likely become protein deficient because rice provides less than 5 percent of usable or complete protein (grams of protein per 100 calories adjusted by quality score or net protein utilization and then expressed in terms of protein calories per 100 total calories), which is the minimum safe level recommended for adults by the World Health Organization. The protein value of beans is about 20 percent usable protein. The combination of rice and beans, however, raises the usable protein value up to 50 percent. This happens because the amino acids in the two foods complement each other. The rice is low in lysine but has a surplus of the sulfur-containing amino acids (e.g., cystine), while conversely the beans are low in the sulfur-containing amino acids, but have a surplus of lysine. Similarly, eating wheat and beans together can increase the protein actually usable by the body by about 33 percent.

Table 2.2. Amino acid strengths and weaknesses of various food groups.

Food Group	Weaknesses	Strengths
Legumes	Tryptophan, Methionine, Cystine*	Lysine, Isoleucine
Grains	Lysine, Isolcucine	Tryptophan, Methionine, Cystine*
Seeds and Nuts	Lysine, Isoleucine (except cashews and pumpkin seeds)	Tryptophan, Methionine, Cystine*
Other Vegetables	Isoleucine, Methionine, Cystine*	Tryptophan, Lysine
Eggs	None	Tryptophan, Lysine, Methionine, Cystine*
Milk Products	None	Lysine

Note: To achieve balanced protein, combine food groups as given in the next table (Table 2.3) so that the amino acid strengths of one compensate for the weaknesses of the other.

*Although cystine is not an essential amino acid, its presence in foods spares methionine, which is essential.

Table 2.3. Typical vegetarian dishes with complete protein.

Grains with Legumes
Rice with Lentils
Macaroni enriched with soy flour
Rice with black-eyed peas
Bean soup with toast
Peanut-butter sandwich
Falafel (chickpea pancake) with pita bread
Bean taco
Grains with Milk
Oatmeal with milk
Macaroni and cheese
Wheat flakes with milk
Cheese sandwich
Rice pudding
Creamed soup with noodles or rice
Pancakes and waffles
Quiche
Breads and muffins made with milk
Meatless lasagna
Granola with milk
Pizza
Legumes with Seeds
Bean curd with sesame seeds
Bean soup with sesame meal
Hummus (chickpea and sesame paste)
Grains with Eggs
Rice pudding
Egg-salad sandwich
Kasha (buckwheat groats)
Noodle pudding
Fried rice

French toast
Oatmeal cookies
Quiche
Other Vegetables with Milk or Eggs
Potato salad
Cheese and potato soup
Mashed potatoes with milk
Vegetable omelet
Eggplant Parmesan
Scalloped potatoes
Broccoli with cheese sauce
Spinach salad with sliced eggs
Cream of pumpkin soup

Table 2.2 shows the amino acid strengths and weaknesses of various food groups, and Table 2.3 lists typical combinations of these various food groups to make dishes with complete protein. As a rule of thumb, keep three simple combinations in mind: (1) combine legumes with grains; (2) combine legumes with nuts and seeds; (3) combine eggs or dairy products with any vegetable protein.

Buddhist monks in Korea who eat an extremely large amount of white rice, 60 percent of their calories, enjoy good health because they supplement their rice with beans and other nutritious food. Many vegetarians in poorer countries are able to survive in good health with no animal food because they get quality protein from combinations of rice and beans or wheat and beans (malnourished vegetarians in poorer countries, however, are due to lack of sufficient food availability). Some food writers such as Frances Lappe (author of a best-seller, *Diet for a Small Planet*, Ballantine Books, New York) suggest beans and rice in the balanced proportion of 1 to 2.7 in order to maximize protein values. However, such precision is not necessary, and vegetarians have enjoyed good health by combining grains and beans to their individual taste for thousands of years.

In most traditional cultures, grains and beans are eaten together in a variety of food combinations. In Mexico, corn tacos and tortillas are eaten with pinto beans. The peasants of Cuba eat rice with black beans. In India, chappatis (flat unleavened whole wheat bread) are eaten with dal (Mung beans, lentils, peas and various other legumes). In China and Japan, tofu (bean curd) is eaten together with rice. Among other combinations that provide good protein values are cereals (grains) and milk, macaroni and cheese, grains and egg (for lacto-ovo-vegetarians), beans and nuts or seeds, and brewer's yeast and grains. To exploit this complementary effect, you can make dishes and plan meals with the help of Tables 2.2 and 2.3 so that the protein in one food fills the amino acid deficiencies in another food.

Obtaining Sufficient Protein Quantity

As for amounts of protein, three things are worth bearing in mind. First, most meat eaters are already consuming twice as much protein as they really need. Second, the protein in milk and eggs is more efficiently used by the body than that in meat, fish, or poultry, so relatively little goes a long way nutritionally. Third, legumes, especially soybeans, contain the largest percentage of protein among vegetable foods and are in the same ballpark as many meats. If legumes play a central role in your diet, you're not likely to shortchange yourself on protein. Thus, one cup of cooked soybeans contains about 20 grams of protein, as much protein as three frankfurters, or 1/4 pound hamburger, or 18 ounces of milk, or 3 ounces of cheese! Each would supply two-thirds of a 60-pound child's daily protein needs, nearly half the recommended protein allowance for a 120-pound adult, and a third the amount needed by a 170-pound man.

In the total diet, nutritionists recommend that protein constitute only 15 percent of your daily calories; fats no more than 30 percent (preferably 10 to 20 percent); and carbohydrates, 55 percent. In cutting back on protein, most Americans will automatically reduce their fat intake, probably to the benefit of their hearts and blood vessels. For example, T-bone steak contains 17% protein and 82%

fat, whereas lentils contain 29% protein and no fat. There is some experimental evidence that too much protein, as well as excess fat, can promote atherosclerosis and cancer (see cancer and heart problems in Chapter 4).

If you are doubtful about adequate consumption of protein, its deficiency can be observed from your body's condition. Because nails, hair, and skin require newly synthesized protein for growth and health, their condition is usually a good indication of whether or not you are getting enough protein. Similarly, notice whether or not abrasions heal quickly. If they don't, you may be seriously lacking protein in your diet. A wholesome diet, followed with understanding of nutritional needs, however, would never lead to this problem.

Considering Calories and Other Nutrients

There is certainly a tendency for vegetarians to have a lower calorie intake than people on non-vegetarian diets. This is largely because, in the absence of meat-eating, vegetarians' fat intake is lower (an advantage in view of the association of high fat consumption with heart disease). However, if higher intake of calories of fat is required, cereal grains contain more than 65 percent carbohydrates and nuts are more than 50 percent fat (see Chapter 5 for nutrient values of vegetarian foods).

The vegetarian diet, with its protein-rich cereals and legumes, is certainly an excellent source of natural vitamins and minerals that people need, and vegetarians tend to have relatively high intakes of calcium, vitamin B, and vitamin C. However, vegetarians living exclusively on vegetables (vegans) have a low dietary intake of two vitamins, B 12 and D. For these people, B 12 tablets can provide extra vitamin B 12 if needed, although for most people on a natural diet, fresh milk and cheese can supplement the diet. However, vitamin B 12 is not needed regularly since it is stored in the liver; the storage supply can last for about 5 years. A deficiency of vitamin B 12 can cause anemia and in extreme cases nervous disorders. Vitamin D is important for the bone development of children, but adults do not generally need vitamin D in their diet. Since it is synthesized under the skin in the presence of sunlight, if one gets enough sunlight, vitamin D deficiency is unlikely. In fact, supplemented milk and margarine supply more than adequate amounts of vitamin D and it has been recommended that fortification of foods other than milk and margarine be reduced or discontinued for the U.S. population.

To assure proper growth and development, infants and young children should include animal protein such as milk and milk products or eggs in their diets. Although a few vegan communities are raising infants according to carefully spelled out vegan nutritional guidelines, in general, this is unadvisable.

Chapter 3

WEIGHT PROBLEMS AND VEGETARIANISM

Weight problems are rare in populations where a lot of natural fruits, vegetables and whole grains are consumed. But excess weight is a common problem in developed countries like the United States, where the progress of scientific and technical development has led to the common consumption of processed and refined foods. One of the obvious effects of this move is the high caloric intake resulting from the decreased volume of processed foods. In other words, over-consumption of calories to fill the stomach, which leads to an overweight problem.

This chapter is intended to introduce the common causes of overweight, the treatments and their limitations, and the effectiveness of fruits, vegetables and whole grains to control this modern day problem. The problem is a new one: never before has man had so wide a choice or so regular a supply of good food and neither did he have such a common use of motor vehicles that even natural exercise such as walking would need special efforts.

Overweight and Its Causes

Overweight or obesity is a condition of the body in which there is an excessive deposit of fat or adipose tissue. (Although most of us know our ideal weight, others can determine this from any standard height and weight table.) Increase of the fat tissue is dependent upon the number (hyperplasia) and size (hypertrophy) of the fat cells (adipocytes), both of which are influenced by variables such as diet and heredity. The early-onset of childhood obesity is frequently accompanied by an increase in the number of fat cells, whereas adult obesity is more commonly accompanied by an increase in the size of fat cells. Studies on adipose tissue or fat cells have led to the following conclusions:

1. Adults, whether normal or obese, have a fixed number of fat

cells in the body, therefore, obesity developing in adult life is associated only with the enlargement of fat cells.

2. Obesity developing in infancy or childhood is associated with an increase in the number of fat cells. Infant-feeding practices which involve high energy intake stimulates an increase in the number of fat cells.

3. Obesity caused by increase in number of fat cells is more resistant to weight-reduction treatment than increase in size of fat cells.

4. The size of the fat cell influences its metabolism. For example, increased insulin resistance in large cells leads to an increase in insulin requirements and a tendency to develop diabetes.

At least one practical lesson is obvious from the above conclusions that early nutrition during childhood does produce an apparent effect on the number of fat cells. Therefore, it is important to introduce youngsters to good eating habits which are nutritionally sound but avoid excessive fat consumption or other excessively high calorie diets. In this way, it is possible to prevent a tendency towards obesity in later life. Higher consumption of carefully selected natural foods as emphasized later in this chapter is one way to introduce children to sound eating habits, which should last a life time. (The lack of exercise does not cause overweight, even though it is important for physical fitness, and has an indirect effect on weight through expending more calories).

What Causes Overweight

Overweight or obesity is generally accepted to be the result of energy intake that is greater than energy expended. In other words, excess weight is the result of an imbalance between energy (measured in calories) consumed as food and energy expended, either in maintaining the basic metabolic processes necessary to sustain life or in performing physical activity. The calories consumed in excess of their use become converted to fat and accumulate in the body as fat, or adipose tissue. It is believed that the rate of fat deposition is higher in overweight people as compared to those with normal weight (due to the effect of overweight on body physiology). Factors which influence obesity and upset the caloric balance may include heredity, endocrine factors, low physical activity of an individual, higher number of fat cells, greater intestinal length, and psychosocial emotional problems. In the psychosocial aspects of over-eating people experience frustration, depression, worry, guilt, shame, hopelessness, isolation and unusual stress which often leads them to seek compensation in eating. To prevent an increase in body weight and body fat because of a caloric imbalance, any program of weight control must establish an equilibrium between energy input and energy output. If you consume more calories than you use, whether from protein, carbohydrate, or fat, you will gain weight. And if you consume fewer calories than you use, you will lose body fat.

Treatments for Overweight and Their Limitations

It is only when the number of calories ingested as food exceeds the daily energy requirements that the excess calories are stored as fat in adipose tissue. Therefore, regardless of the cause of overweight (such as genetic make-up or poor eating habits), there are two ways to lose weight: (a) either cut down food calories taken in (the dietary control of weight), or (b) raise the number of calories expended as energy, through physical activity.

The dietary control of weight, however, is more effective and should contain a program that provides a permanent solution to your weight problem. As you may have noticed, many popular books or articles on exotic diets or exercise plans usually claim their plans to be easy and effortless to follow. If this were the case, then millions of adults and teenagers who are overweight could be cured easily.

> **Note**: A calorie is the unit used for measuring the heat
> or energy producing value of food when it is burned
> by the body. In the diet, a calorie describes the

amount of energy potentially available in a given food. It is also used to describe the amount of energy the body must use up to perform a given function. The caloric value of a specific food depends on the composition of the food in terms of protein, fat and carbohydrate. When the average efficiency of digestion is taken into account, the net caloric value for proteins and carbohydrates is 4 calories per 1 gram of protein or carbohydrate, and for fat is 9 calories per 1 gram of fat.

Generally, exotic diets produce a weight loss primarily due to loss of body water during the first several weeks. Unless a person can maintain a reduced caloric intake for a considerable time, the weight will eventually be regained. The net result is a return to original body size, often at the expense of feelings of hunger and other psychological stresses while the diet plan is actually followed. In fact, people who live from one best-selling weight-loss scheme to the next, often end up with rhythmic loss and gain patterns of weight. Studies indicate that the repeated gaining, losing, and regaining of extra pounds is more damaging to physical health than just remaining overweight. That's why it's so important to forget all the gimmicks, the crash programs and diets you could not possibly follow for long, and find instead a permanent solution to your weight problem.

If you have already tried one of the weight loss programs and failed, you are not alone. It may be reassuring to know that most of these weight loss programs (according to the statistics obtained by a review of the scientific literature) do not provide permanent solutions because sooner or later most of the people discontinue the program and return to old, eating habits that made them obese in the first place.

Some of the common weight loss practices include fad diets, formula diets, fasting or starvation, calorie-restricted diets or physical activity, which are effective only to a certain degree for various lengths of time, many of these at the cost of a physical as well as psychological health loss. The permanent and painless solution to an overweight problem is a change of eating habits, and even more important is the addition of wholesome vegetarian foods as discussed in this chapter.

Treating an Overweight Problem with Vegetarian Diet

The effectiveness of a wholesome vegetarian diet in weight control could be due to several reasons. First of all, vegetarian diets are simply low in calories and saturated fat but high in health promoting minerals and vitamins. Secondly, the fiber content in vegetarian foods gives the dieter a feeling of fullness in the stomach, which reduces the appetite. Studies on high fiber diets also claim that it requires more chewing. Chewing (mastication) diminishes the sensation of abnormal appetite that compels a person to eat more than is needed. This results in a diet that responds only to natural hunger. It is possible that because of the decrease in bowel transit time caused by the high fiber content of natural foods, small amounts of the fat and protein you eat are excreted. Therefore, a few of the calories you eat really don't count. A high fiber content may also inhibit absorption of nutrients through the intestine, thus encouraging weight loss. Although some of the nutrients not absorbed may be categorized as "essential," the consumption of protein and other nutrients by most Americans is so much in excess of what is needed that this degree of loss is not likely to be a problem.

Considering the overweight problem and weight-consciousness of Americans, however, it is surprising that more people have not become vegetarians. Perhaps lack of awareness about vegetarian nutrition and cooking has been a major contributing factor. As you see, vegetables are very low in calories and high in health-promoting natural minerals and vitamins; and their bulk fills the stomach and thus satisfies the appetite. For example, 5 ounces of meat provides 500 calories, whereas the same amount of cooked kidney beans provides only 167 calories. Green beans and other fresh vegetables are even lower in calories, and on the average provide less than one fourth of the calories provided by kidney beans. A lunch of vegetable soup, a slice of whole-grain bread, and a cottage cheese and fruit salad has a third fewer calories than a cheeseburger lunch (and far, far less saturated fat and cholesterol). And for the caloric value of a 6-ounce steak, a vegetarian could eat 3 cups of rice or a whole pound of noodles or, to be more reasonable, the vegetarian could eat a very generous serving of a casserole of noodles, vegetables, and cheese, which would eliminate the need for the potatoes and carrots in the steak dinner. A meal of a cup of brown rice and lentils, two slices of whole-grain bread (or a large baked potato) with margarine, 1/2 cup each of carrots and peas, a lettuce and tomato salad with dressing, and a fruit salad containing a banana, one apple, one orange, 2 tablespoons of raisins, and half a dozen walnuts, would contain about 890 calories (610 less than the steak dinner) and leave the diner positively stuffed. While this is not typical of a meal that might be prepared by an experienced vegan, it does illustrate the huge amounts of food a vegan can consume without exceeding the body's caloric needs.

According to the diet philosophy presented here, it is not necessary to become a food crank and weigh, measure, and analyze every mouthful of food. It is simply true that you are unlikely to grow fat by including good amounts of fresh vegetables and fruits in your diet. Most of these are over 80 percent water and contain only the merest traces of fat and very little carbohydrate. A group of young vegetarians studied in Boston weighed an average 33 pounds less than a meat-eating comparison group, because as mentioned earlier, a vegetarian diet is bulky and filling, and it's hard to eat more calories than your body burns. As a result, most people lose weight when they start a vegetarian diet. Those who are strict vegetarians (vegans) and eat no dairy products or eggs may actually have a hard time consuming enough calories to maintain their weight. Clearly, for an obese person a vegetarian diet with its naturally lower caloric content is a blessing. However, a normal (or underweight) person does need to make some adjustments in both total food intake and intake of adequate amounts of foods such as legumes, cereals and nuts to add calories for achieving an appropriate caloric balance.

To suit the wide range of tastes and dietary habits of Westerners, meat analogues may be included to replace meat until you start enjoying exclusively vegetarian foods. Meat analogues are made with soybeans, molded into common meat foods such as sausages and burgers. Even if you are not a vegetarian, you may find some of the analogues to be attractive, economical, and healthy alternatives to meat.

Even if you have no interest in vegetarianism, there's no reason why you should have animal protein at every meal or even every day. By including vegetarian dishes in your daily menu and adapting the vegetarian approach to menu planning, you can greatly reduce your dependence on animal protein and especially on high-fat, high-calorie meats.

Natural Diet Plan to Getting Thin and Staying Thin, Feel Healthy but not Hungry

As you know from the preceding pages, the natural diet containing whole foods of plant origin (except milk) is generally low in fat, cholesterol and caloric values, but high in stomach-filling bulk such as fiber, and in health promoting natural vitamins and minerals. The following pages will include diet plans mainly as guidelines. Although these are confined for the most part to natural vegetarian foods, fat free lean meats and meat analogues (discussed in preceding section) may be included in small amounts as a supplement until you start enjoying exclusively vegetarian foods.

To follow the diet plan you can easily improvise you own menu for the day from the listed food groups (Table 3.1). As a rule of thumb, include foods from the first three groups varying from 1 to 4 servings depending on individual weight status. Table 3.1 provides an example of how to select various food groups to choose a diet of 1,000 calories which provides 53 grams of protein. For maximum weight loss with an intake of 600-700 calories, choose one serving from group 1 and two from each of groups 2 and 3. From the vegetable and fruit groups 4 and 5 choose about 4 servings. In fact, the foods from groups 4, 5 and 6 are so low calorically that they can be eaten in relatively unlimited amounts. To keep from being hungry these unrestricted foods help the dieter avoid the temptation to deviate by providing a satisfying sense of bulk while adding very few calories.

Unless there is a serious weight problem, weighing of food is not necessary as long as you are eating plenty of natural food, particularly from groups 4 and 5 with the added taste of seasonings from group 6. As you may notice, the fat food group is not added. In addition to the natural fat provided by the foods themselves, most of the cooking requires frying in vegetable oils such as corn, cottonseed, safflower, soy, sunflower, olive and margarine which will provide enough fat.

A variety of vegetables (for vegetarian recipes see Dhillon, Health, *Happiness and Longevity: Eastern and Western Approach.* Japan Publications, Tokyo/ Harper & Row, New York, 1983. If not available, in printed edition, you can buy digital edition at Amazon or Barnes & Noble in e-Book format.) can lead you to new, interesting, low-calorie dishes of excellent taste which can keep you slim and healthy for the rest of your life. However, cooking vegetables requires a great deal of time in preparation for peeling, slicing, chopping, etc. You can cut down the time by cooking extra quantities for the freezer. Unlike many diet books, sample menus are not provided here (an example of menus as a guideline, however, is given in appendix B). Taste is a personal choice and, perhaps like you, I do not like someone to tell me what to eat. As long as you follow the guidelines to include foods from all the six groups mentioned in Table 3.1 with special emphasis on groups 4 and 5, you do not have to count calories or follow any sample menus. Compulsively counting calories and rigidly following sample menus of foods you do not like is not a part of the natural vegetarian diet philosophy.

NOTE: "Health, Happiness & Longevity" as well as other books mentioned in this book or listed on page 2 are available at Amazon, Barnes & Noble and other book sellers.

Table 3.1. Example for selecting a 1000 calorie diet from various food groups.

Food Group	Approx. serving size	No. of servings	Calories	Protein (g)	Carbohy-drates(g)	Fat (g)
1. Dairy Products (non-fat)	1 cup	2	160	16	24	-
2. Grains and starchy Vegetables	1 slice or 1/2 cup	4	280	8	60	-
3. Legumes	1/2 CUP	3	300	21	60	5
4. Vegetables	1/2 CUP	No limit (4)	100	8	20	-
5. Fruits	Equiv.1 apple	No limit (4)	160	-	40	-
6. Beverages and	As desired	No limit	0	-	-	-
		Total	**1,000**	**53**	**204**	**5**

NOTE: For more information on Weight Control, please see our guide **"A Simple Solution to America's Weight Problem."**

Chapter 4

VEGETARIANISM IN HEALTH AND DISEASE

A vegetarian diet can be used as a medicine chiefly in the preventive sense by eating food in its natural state as much as possible. It is believed that many ailments are caused by accumulation of poison through improper eating and that a steady intake of selected foods fortifies the body against various health problems. For example, sinus congestion has been associated with an over-consumption of mucus and acid-forming foods; replacing fruits and vegetables for milk and meat should relieve congestion problems. Freshly made vegetable and fruit juices are very good for those who suffer from chronic ailments, yet raw vegetable juices should not be thought of as a drug to cure ailments. They are rather the most vital rebuilding and regenerating foods that the body can use for construction. If one intends to feed only on freshly made juice for a week or two, one can drink several pints of juice a day. At times one can feel discomfort from feeding on raw juices, usually because of the stirring up of toxins accumulated in the system, but soon energy and vigor return when the toxins are eliminated. Dr. John Harvey Kellog (of the family that started the cereal company), Medical Director, Battle Creek (Michigan) Sanitarium, used fruits, cereals, and fresh vegetables to make an "antitoxic diet" for his patients.

As stated above, such preventive uses of vegetarian diets may seem a thin basis for avoiding or reducing meat and adopting a vegetarian diet today; however, various healthy effects of vegetarian diets are being uncovered by recent scientific findings. For example, a vegetarian diet that reduces the consumption of meat and animal fat and provides high fiber content has been shown to be beneficial against problems related to heart, cancer, uric acid and the digestive system. Many of these are discussed below.

High-fiber Food in the Vegetarian Diet and the Role of Fiber in Health

Wholesome natural food eaten raw provides an excellent source of roughage or fiber which is often lacking in processed food and meat. The importance of fiber in health has become so obvious that nutritionists can no longer avoid paying attention to its role.

Fiber is the cell wall material of plants which adds roughage or bulk to our food; and it is not digestible except for small amounts broken down by intestinal bacteria. Chemically it is made up of cellulose, hemicellulose, lignin, pectin, and cutin. The quantity of each constituent depends on the specific plant and may vary within each species. The most common sources of fiber in our diets are whole grains, fruits, and vegetables. Table 4.1 gives fiber content in some common foods.

Table 4.1 Dietary fiber content of some common foods.

Food	Approx. Measure	Weight (grams)	Fiber (grams)	Fiber (%)
GRAINS				
All-bran or 100% bran	1 cup	70	23.0	33
Bran buds	3 /4 cup	60	18.0	30
Cracked wheat (bulgar), dry	1/3 cup	50	5.6	11
Grapenuts	1/3 cup	45	5.0	11
Grits, dry	1/4 cup	45	4.8	11
Rice, brown, cooked	1 cup	65	1.1	2
Rice, white, cooked	1 cup	65	0.4	1
Rolled oats, dry	1/2 cup	50	4.5	9
Rye bread	1 slice	25	2.0	8
Rye crackers	3 wafers	20	2.3	12
Shredded wheat	2 biscuits	50	6.1	12
Whole-wheat bread	1 slice	25	2.4	10
FRUITS				
Apple	1 small	90	3.1	3

Banana	1 medium	100	1.8	2
Cantaloupe, cube	3 /4 cup	120	1.4	1
Cherries, raw	10	70	0.8	1
Grapefruit	1/2	200	2.6	1
Grapes, raw	16	60	0.4	1
Orange	1 small	90	1.8	2
Peach, raw	1 medium	100	1.3	1
Peaches, canned, slices	1/2 cup	120	1.3	1
Pear, raw	1 medium	120	2.8	2
Pears, canned	1/2 cup	125	1.4	1
Plum, raw	2 small	9	1.6	18
Strawberries	1/2 cup	125	2.6	2
Tangerine	1 medium	10	2.1	21
VEGETABLES				
Beans, green	1/2 cup	50	1.2	2
Beets, cooked	1/3 cup	100	2.1	2
Broccoli, cooked	3/4 cup	75	1.6	2
Cabbage, cooked	3/4 cup	100	2.2	2
Cabbage, raw	1 cup	75	2.1	3
Carrots, cooked	3/4 cup	100	2.1	2
Carrots, raw	1 medium	100	3.7	4

Cauliflower, cooked	1/2 cup	100	1.2	1
Cauliflower, raw	1 cup	100	1.8	2
Celery, cooked	2/3 cup	100	2.4	2
Celery, raw	2½ stalks	100	3.0	3
Corn kernels	2/3 cup	110	4.2	4
Cucumber	1/2 of 7 inch	100	1.5	2
Kale, cooked	1/2 cup	100	2.0	2
Kidney beans, cooked	1 cup	100	2.0	2
Lentils, cooked	1/2 cup	100	4.0	4
Lettuce	1cup	50	0.8	2
Parsnips, cooked	3/4 cup	120	5.9	5
Peas, cooked	1/2 cup	60	3.8	6
Potatoes, cooked	2/3 cup	90 (raw)	3.1	3
Spinach	2 large leaves	50	1.8	4
Summer squash, cooked	1/2 cup	100	2.2	2
Summer squash, raw	1 5- inch	100	3.0	3
Turnips, raw	1 cup	100	2.2	2

SOURCE: Based on analyses of Dr. J. W. Anderson, University of Kentucky Medical Center, Lexington, Kentucky.

The role of fiber in our health is quite well-accepted by the scientific community. Fiber has been shown to prevent common noninfective diseases of the colon, such as constipation, diverticulosis (a disease in which little pouches form along the intestinal tract but most frequently in the colon), and cancer (see next section). Fiber affects, stool bulk, softness, and transit time. It has been theorized that a high-fiber diet, by cutting bowl transit time, allows less time for bacteria in the colon to produce carcinogens (cancer-producing substances). Rural Ugandans who hardly ever get cancer of the colon, eat considerable fiber. Their average bowel transit time is 36 hours, compared to 77 hours for British men who consumed lower-fiber diets like most Americans. Although cancer of the colon has also been claimed to be related to fat consumption, this does not eliminate the possibility that fiber plays a role in the disease. A high-fiber diet may also protect against a variety of other diseases including heart disease (by lowering blood cholesterol), appendicitis, gallstones, hemorrhoids and diabetes.

The findings about the role of dietary fiber in lowering blood cholesterol are among the most encouraging for heart patients. The types of fiber which have beneficial effects are the ones consumed from natural foods, but not bran. Bran is more than 90 percent cellulose and has no beneficial effect on cholesterol levels. Pectins (found in most fruits), guar gum (found in beans), and the fiber in rolled oats and carrots are especially useful in lowering blood cholesterol. When patients were given 5 grams of guar gum before each meal, cholesterol dropped an average of 10.6 percent over and above the reduction caused by the drugs. Scottish researchers showed that eating 7 ounces of raw carrots at breakfast every day for three weeks could reduce the cholesterol level by 11 percent and increase the amount of fat excreted by 50 percent. Fiber's cholesterol lowering effect may result from its ability to increase the excretion of bile acids, which are made from cholesterol. Physiologists at the University of Southampton in England showed that the fiber consumed by vegetarians can lower blood pressure.

The influence of fiber on blood-sugar levels and insulin requirements is another beneficial effect of dietary fiber. By including fiber in their diets, Dr. J.W. Anderson, V.A. Hospital, Lexington, Kentucky, found that some diabetics have been able to get along without insulin or other antidiabetic medication. Here, too, pectin and guar gum are the most effective plant fibers. Another popular plus for fiber is that it encourages weight loss (see chapter 3).

As for how much fiber you should eat, no one can yet say. Vegetarians, however, should not be concerned. The studies have shown that on average vegetarians get over 50 percent more fiber than meat eaters. Non-vegetarians and those who consume excessive amounts of processed foods and refined grains are likely to have lower fiber consumption. They do not need to buy a jar of fiber pills or boxes of bran and pectin, all they need to do is to increase consumption of wholesome vegetarian foods. In fact, calculating the amount of fiber consumed is not necessary, but including whole grain foods, fresh fruits, and vegetables in the diet should be the main concern. Since fiber is relatively hard to digest and may also cause excessive intestinal gas problems, a steady increase of fiber from natural foods only, without the use of added fiber, is advisable; these problems, however, are temporary and subside in a few weeks when the bacterial population of your digestive system adapts to increased fiber intake.

Importance of a Vegetarian Diet in Regularity

The ability of fibrous vegetarian foods to counter the problem of constipation has long been known to the medical profession and the general public. In the United States alone more than 700 different laxative preparations are sold over the counter, and one percent of all prescriptions are for laxatives. Many of these drugs act as stimulants to the colon, and their repeated use can lead to a chronic inability of the colon to act on its own. These drugs may also cause cramps, diarrhea, and excessive loss of fluids and essential minerals. The sensible way to treat constipation, therefore, is to consume wholesome vegetarian foods, and not to use laxative drugs.

The fiber from wholesome vegetarian foods absorbs lots of water, softening the stool, increasing its volume, and making it easier to pass, and it speeds the elimination of food wastes. Apples, fresh carrots, and cabbage are useful in countering constipation, as are bulk laxatives like Metamucil (hemicellulose and gum extracted from psyllium seeds). However, Dr. Peter Van Soest, nutrition researcher at Cornell University, has shown that although coarse bran and cellulose have a laxative effect, finely ground bran and wood cellulose that may be bought as a fine fiber induces constipation. Therefore, the increase of fiber from wholesome vegetarian foods only, without the use of added fiber, is advisable to counter the constipation and other problems related to low fiber intake.

Your stools are the best indicators of healthy eating habits. The healthier stools should show the following characteristics:
1. These should be lighter in weight. See whether the stools float or sink down in the toilet. If they float, you're eating the right kind of foods. Fiber from foods makes them float.
2. There should be no offensive smell, more than mild odor.
3. The offensive smell is not natural. It's indication of wrong foods and wrong microbes occupying your digestive system.

Importance of Vegetarian Diet against Cancer

That diet plays a part in causing human cancer is suggested by the following statistical observations: (1) the differing rates of cancer incidence in different countries with different eating habits; (2) the altered rates of cancer occurrence in migrants from a country with a low rate of a particular cancer to one with a high rate of such cancer, and vice versa; (3) the cancer rates in populations with particular dietary habits; and (4) the time trends of cancer incidence. Most persuasive are the sharp differences in cancer rates between Japan and the U.S., where fat, mostly of animal origin, accounts for 40 to 50 percent of calories in the U.S. and only 10 to 20 percent in Japan.

The diets with positive effect on cancer control are the ones that provide fiber, vitamin C, vitamin A, and vegetables from the cabbage (crucifer) family. The diet high in fat and cholesterol on the other hand contributes to various cancers.

Research findings during the last decade have revealed that the diet high in animal fats and cholesterol contributes to the growth of cancers of the colon, breast, and uterus. For example, among the Seventh-Day Adventists, most of whom eat no meat or poultry, these cancers are quite rare, but they are leading cancers among other meat-eating Americans. There are several possible explanations for this relationship between diet and cancers. With regard to colon cancer, diets rich in saturated fats and cholesterol may result in large accumulations of natural cancer-promoting chemicals in the gut. And the relatively low fiber content of such diets may result in slow-moving bowels and prolonged contact of the cancer-promoting chemicals with body tissues (see also the section on role of fiber in health). Therefore, it is possible that the risk of colon cancer could be lessened by consuming less fat and more fiber as suggested by the American Health Foundation. As for cancers of the breast and uterus, their growth is stimulated by estrogen hormones. A non-vegetarian diet high in fat and cholesterol results in the production of estrogen-like hormones in the gut, and similar hormones are produced in fatty tissue that forms excessive body fat. Once developed, whether a low-fat diet will slow down the growth or spread of breast or uterus cancer remains to be shown. The better survival of breast cancer patients in Japan (10-20 percent fat calories) compared with the United States (40-50 percent fat calories) would suggest that a low fat diet may be of some benefit.

In addition to the above explanations for reduced risk of cancer among vegetarians, a variety of vegetable foods and fruit, including brussels sprouts, cauliflower, broccoli, turnips, cabbage, spinach, celery, citrus fruits, beans, and seeds, can stimulate the production of anticancer enzymes in the body. Dr. Saxon Graham, Professor of Social and Preventive Medicine at State University of New York, found that chemicals in vegetables belonging to the cabbage family block the action of certain cancer-causing substances. In addition to the contribution of fiber, vitamin A, C or E by these vegetables, this happens through the enhancement of aryl hydrocarbon hydroxylase (AHH) activity by indoles in these plants. (Another set of hypotheses deals with the ingestion of vitamin A foods such as green vegetables that decrease the risk of cancer, such as lung cancer among heavy smokers). Low fat, low protein, higher fiber, and the presence of anticancer enzymes in vegetarian foods has also been associated with a decrease in risk for several other kinds of cancers like pancreatic and prostate cancer. In view of these observations, the consumption of grains, vegetables and fruits as mentioned above should reduce the chances of developing cancer.

Vegetarian Diet can Help Against Heart Problems

A comparative study of diet and, heart disease in seven countries showed that the Finns, who consumed the most animal fats, also had the highest death rate. Americans were next, but the Greeks and Italians, who eat relatively little animal fat, were near the bottom of the heart disease death rate list. In Japan, where very little fat of any kind is eaten, the heart disease death rate is lower than in any other industrialized nation, despite high rates of high blood pressure and cigarette smoking. In America, Seventh-Day Adventists, most of whom eat no meat or poultry, have only 60 percent the amount of heart diseases as compared to other Americans. In Boston a study of 116 vegetarians showed that they had lower blood pressures and cholesterol levels than comparable groups of meat-eating young adults. But those vegetarians who consumed dairy products and eggs more than five times a week had higher blood pressures and cholesterol levels than those who ate these animal foods less often or not at all.

Even those vegetarians who eat dairy products and eggs, which contain saturated animal fat and cholesterol, are not likely to come anywhere near the fat and cholesterol content of the typical mixed American diet. Conventional American meals make excessive meat eating almost inevitable; there is a substantial amount of fat in most of the meat and only a small proportion of it is polyunsaturated. Saturated fats (mostly from animal origin or hydrogenated fat) in human diets influence amounts of plasma lipids and serum cholesterol. Increased levels of both cholesterol and lipids results in hardening of the arteries which causes such vascular disorders as hypertension or high blood pressure. By substituting saturated with highly unsaturated fats (e.g., from safflower, corn and cotton seed oil), the amount of plasma lipid and serum cholesterol is lowered. The removal of both saturated as well as unsaturated fats from the diet is even more effective in lowering blood cholesterol. In fact, the influence of fat on increasing serum cholesterol is much more effective than direct dietary intake of cholesterol. Lowered consumption of fat, particularly the saturated fat of meat origin, therefore, can reduce considerably the risks of lipid and cholesterol related heart problems. Furthermore, vegetarian diets not only reduce the intake of animal fat and cholesterol but also increase the intake of dietary fiber that has been associated with reduction of cholesterol levels and related heart problems as discussed in the earlier section on fiber.

Vegetarian Diet May Cut Cholesterol As Much As Drugs Do:

Results published in the Journal of the American Medical Association (July 23, 2003) indicate that a strict low-fat vegetarian diet high in specific plant products can lower levels of bad cholesterol as much as widely-prescribed statin drugs can.

The diet that produced these study results was a strict vegetarian diet that included certain foods (eggplant, soy, almonds, barley, okra, etc.) that have already proven to control cholesterol levels. David J. A. Jenkins of the University of Toronto and his colleagues tested a specific vegetarian diet that combined many of these food groups into one menu that contained high amounts of plant sterols, fiber, nuts and soy protein. Of the 46 patients with high cholesterol levels that the team studied, 16 ate this diet for a month. A second group of 16 ate a regular low-fat vegetarian diet and 14 participants consumed the low-fat diet and took 20 milligrams of lovastatin, a standard cholesterol-reducing drug. At the end of the study period, those patients who ate the special diet lowered their levels of LDL cholesterol (the "bad" type associated with clogging coronary arteries) by 29 percent whereas the patients taking lovastatin reduced their LDL levels by 31 percent. The low-fat dieters, in contrast, showed just an 8 percent decrease in the amount of LDL present. "As we age, we tend to get raised cholesterol, which in turn increases our risk of heart disease," Jenkins explains. "This study shows that people now have a dietary alternative to drugs to control their cholesterol, at least initially."

Although more studies will need to be done to backup the link between a veggie diet and healthy cholesterol researchers are optimistic that they may be on a roadway toward a drugless therapy for lowering cholesterol that will benefit many individuals.

Low fat veggie diet best bet for treating diabetes

A low-fat vegetarian diet treats type 2 diabetes more effectively than a standard diabetes diet and may be more effective than single-agent therapy with oral diabetes drugs, according to a study in the August, 2006 issue of Diabetes Care, a journal published by the American Diabetes Association.

Study participants on the low-fat vegan diet showed dramatic improvement in four disease markers: blood sugar control, cholesterol reduction, weight control, and kidney function.

The randomized controlled trial was conducted by doctors and dieticians with the Physicians Committee for Responsible Medicine (PCRM), the George Washington University, and the University of Toronto with funding from the National Institutes of Health and the Diabetes Action Research and Education Foundation.

The vegan diet represents a major departure from current diabetes diets, in that it placed no limits on calories, carbohydrates, or portions. "The diet appears remarkably effective, and all the side effects are good ones--especially weight loss and lower cholesterol," says lead researcher Neal D. Barnard, M.D., PCRM president and adjunct associate professor of medicine at the George Washington University. "I hope this study will rekindle interest in using diet changes first, rather than prescription drugs."

Vegetables may keep brains young

New research on vegetables and aging found that eating vegetables appears to help keep the brain young and may slow the mental decline sometimes associated with growing old.

On measures of mental sharpness, older people who ate more than two servings of vegetables daily appeared about five years younger at the end of the six-year study than those who ate few or no vegetables.

The research in almost 2,000 Chicago-area men and women doesn't prove that vegetables reduce mental decline, but it adds to mounting evidence pointing in that direction. The findings also echo previous research in women only.

Green leafy vegetables including spinach, kale and collards appeared to be the most beneficial. The researchers said that may be because they contain healthy amounts of vitamin E, an antioxidant that is believed to help fight chemicals produced by the body that can damage cells.

Vegetables generally contain more vitamin E than fruits, which were not linked with slowed mental decline in the study. Vegetables also are often eaten with healthy fats such as salad oils, which help the body absorb vitamin E and other antioxidants, said lead author Martha Clare Morris, a researcher at the Rush Institute for Healthy Aging at Chicago's Rush University Medical Center.

The fats from healthy oils can help keep cholesterol low and arteries clear, which both contribute to brain health.

The study was published in the October, 2006 issue of the journal Neurology and funded with grants from the National Institute on Aging.

"This is a sound paper and contributes to our understanding of cognitive decline," said Dr. Meir Stampfer of Harvard's School of Public Health.

"The findings specific for vegetables and not fruit add further credibility that this is not simply a marker of a more healthful lifestyle," said Stampfer, who was not involved in the research.

The research involved 1,946 people aged 65 and older who filled out questionnaires about their eating habits. A vegetable serving equaled about a half-cup chopped or one cup if the vegetable was a raw leafy green like spinach.

They also had mental function tests three times over about six years; about 60 percent of the study volunteers were black.

The tests included measures of short-term and delayed memory, which asked these older people to recall elements of a story that had just been read to them. The participants also were given a flashcard-like exercise using symbols and numbers.

Overall, people did gradually worse on these tests over time, but those who ate more than two vegetable servings a day had about 40 percent less mental decline than those who ate few or no vegetables. Their test results resembled what would be expected in people about five years younger, Morris said.

The study also found that people who ate lots of vegetables were more physically active, adding to evidence that "what's good for your heart is good for your brain," said neuroscientist Maria Carillo, director of medical and scientific relations for the Alzheimer's Association.

Vegetarian Diet and Longevity

Getting older is inevitable, but the food can slow down the aging process. What we eat can make a difference in how the body ages. Research on the role of foods and aging is still in early stages but at this point the best route to take seems to be focusing on vegetarian foods - increase your fruits, vegetables, and whole grains. In addition to the benefits these foods provide, some nuts, and plenty of water also seem to help maintain health and fight disease which translates into longevity.

The role of plant foods in disease prevention, and the slowing of the aging process, appears to rest with the phytochemicals (plant compounds) that they contain. Phytochemicals function in one of four different ways: (1) These act as antioxidants which work to remove or block the changes in cells that cause disease and aging. (2) These act as detoxifiers, which help the body destroy or eliminate toxic compounds. (3) These act as Hormone regulators by acting as hormones, which produce specific effect on the activity of cells remote from their points of origin. (4) These phytochemicals also function as cell regulators. Cell regulators control the rampant cell growth of tumors, thus protecting against some cancers. Most plant foods contain a variety of phytochemicals making most of them good choices for a variety of ailments. One way to judge the presence of phytochemicals is to look for darkly colored or strong flavored fruits and vegetables. Broccoli, kale, cabbage, brussels sprouts and cauliflower help fight colon cancer and may help with estrogen metabolism.

Here is a glimpse of foods that can help with different body functions: Blueberries, cranberries, cherries and strawberries help fight heart disease, urinary tract infection and may help older adults improve balance, coordination and short-term memory. Spinach, along with kale, broccoli and Brussels sprouts have been found to decrease the incidence of cataracts and macular degeneration, the leading causes of blindness in people over 50. Strawberries, kiwi and plums also seem to help with improved balance, coordination and short-term memory in studies in rats; whether these results will transfer to humans isn't clear, but scientists feel it is likely that they will. Soy protein, blackberries, raspberries, scallions and garlic aid cholesterol reduction, and the list goes on

Walnuts, and flaxseed contain a type of fat called Omega 3, which is associated with a reduction in risk for macular degeneration. Omega-3 fatty acids are also known for their positive effect on reducing Triglycerides (another type of blood fat) and for making blood less sticky and less likely to clot. Thus help with reducing heart attacks or strokes. This same blood thinning effect may help blood vessels in the eyes.

Water is important to cell health and function. Staying well hydrated is important as we age, since the recognition of thirst diminishes with age.

The best advice to prevent the maladies of old age is to try eight to ten servings of fruits and vegetables everyday. Here are some more tips:

a. Make sure the fruits and vegetables are a variety of dark, deep colors and/or strong flavors.
b. Choose whole grain breads, cereals and pasta the majority of the time.
c. Limit dairy food to fat free kinds.
d. Use simple sugars (candies, table sugar, jams, etc) in small amounts and only after including all the fruits, vegetables and whole grains.
e. Stay well hydrated by using at least 64 ounces of water or other water based beverage everyday.

Sometimes all the best intentions still don't get the right foods into our eating plan, this is where - supplements maybe needed, but add supplements only after checking with your physician and/or dietitian. Some supplements may interfere with other medication you're taking. In addition the research on supplements, their safety and long term benefits is still in the very early stages of research; you want to add what might help but won't hurt.

Vitamin and mineral supplements are different and often are important. If you can't get the calcium your bones need or if you're struggling to get the produce you need, a multi vitamin will put the vitamins and minerals back, but not the phytochemicals or the protein and carbohydrate that come from wholesome vegetarian foods. Remember supplement means adds to, not use in place of, so always try for the foods first.

For more information on longevity see our guide: *"Forever Young."*

Vegetarian Diet against Other Unhealthy Effects

The various unhealthy effects of a diet high in meat have been uncovered by recent scientific findings. A diet high in meat, for example, is suggested as a contributing factor in uric acid diseases. A pound of liver contains 19 grains of uric acid and a pound of beefsteak 14 grains, whereas the amount of uric acid the body produces and eliminates through the kidneys daily is only about 6 grains. As a person's liver and kidneys are not able to deal with the extra intake, the uneliminated uric acid becomes the seedbed of gout, rheumatism, headaches, epilepsy, convulsions, nervousness, etc.

The common problem of premenstrual syndrome (PMS) among women is affected by food, because it influences the female hormone level. Foods that help to relieve the trouble are surprisingly wholesome health foods of plant origin. Whole grain (breads, cereals), vegetables, fruits, and safflower oil are among the good ingredients. Foods that worsen the problem are steak, chocolate chip cookies, pretzels and other foods with salt and sugar, and among drinks are wine and coffee.

Among other problems are gallstones that may cause severe abdominal pain. These are more frequently encountered in the developed nations than in the less advanced countries. We do not know with certainty the environmental factors that influence the risk of gallstones; however, it is widely believed that the lack of fiber or roughage, and the excess food cholesterol or fat in the diet are involved. The vegetarian diets with low sugar and high-fiber also help to reduce risks of hypoglycemia or low blood sugar problems. The list could go on, but the bottom line is that by increasing the amount of whole grains, fresh fruits, and vegetables in our diet, we can safely avoid many of the health and life threatening diseases.

Chapter 5

VEGETARIAN FOODS FOR HEALTH

Vegetarianism is an alternative that can offer a surprisingly tasty and varied diet which can be nutritionally sound. In addition it also saves money. With proper cooking the taste of vegetables can be more enjoyable than that of fat-saturated bacon and hot dogs. Choose vegetables and fruits of your choice and make them a major part of your daily meals. Avoid the saturated fats and concentrated proteins of meat origin; satisfy your protein needs by selecting legumes such as soybeans along with cereals and milk for obtaining all the amino acids.

The importance given to meat in western diets is curious considering that the choice of meat is limited to beef, lamb, pork, chicken and fish --only a minority of people venture beyond these. By comparison, plants can give an infinite variety of natural flavors to a diet, without the need for elaborate artifice by the cook. Provided a vegetarian knows about protein sources, there are a wide variety of vegetarian foods that can replace the protein supplied in a non-vegetarian diet by meat, fish and poultry.

Our thinking about the need for huge amounts of animal protein is changing as we are learning that an overabundance of animal protein actually can be detrimental to health. Without a doubt, vegetables rank high among the good ingredients of a diet; what is required is a reasonably good knowledge about vegetarian foods. If you choose your foods properly, you will not have to take any vitamin or mineral supplements. Good nutrition is always balanced and complete, but we don't have to be biochemists or nutritionists to keep our diets balanced. The simple and easy way is to include each of these four groups of foods in the daily menu: (1) bread and cereal group (four servings), (2) protein group--legumes and nuts (two servings), (3) fruit-vegetable group (four servings), (4) milk group (two, three or four servings for adults, children and teens, respectively). (For approximate serving size, see Table 3.1 in chapter 3.)

Bread and Cereal Group

Cereal grains furnish the bulk of the world food supply. The six main crops--wheat, rice, rye, oats, corn and barley--would provide enough grain, if shared out equally today, for each person in the world to have nearly six hundred pounds (270 kg) a year. Cereal and cereal products are high in carbohydrates and furnish approximately 50 percent of the calories consumed by the people of the world. The nutritional composition of various cereal grains is listed in Table 5.1. A cereal grain consists of three parts: the inner germ, the protective endosperm, and the outer bran layer. The germ or embryo of the grain is one of the best sources of thiamin and vitamin E. It also contains B-complex vitamins, fat, minerals (especially iron), carbohydrate and complete protein. Endosperm makes up approximately 85 percent of the grain and is chiefly carbohydrate, with some protein in the form of gluten. The bran or outer layer is chiefly cellulose (fiber) plus B-complex vitamins and minerals, especially iron. Whole grains include all three parts and provide significant amounts of iron, thiamin, riboflavin and niacin. Highly refined cereal grain products contain only the endosperm, and lack fiber and natural minerals and vitamins. The consumption of whole grain products is, therefore, highly important to obtain the high nutritional value of the bread and cereal group.

Table 5.1. Comparative (%) amounts of nutrients in various foods.

Percent Of							
Food Source	Protein	Carbo-hydrate	Fat	Vitamins and Minerals	Fiber	Water	Calories per 100g (3.5 ounces)
Cereal Grain							
Barley	8.00	75.00	1.50	2.00	1.50	12.00	350
Corn and Millet	11.00	69.00	4.50	2.00	1.50	12.00	350
Oats	11.50	66.00	9.00	2.00	1.50	10.00	400
Rice	7.00	76.50	1.00	2.00	1.50	12.00	360
Rye	7.50	72.00	2.00	2.00	1.50	15.00	330

Wheat	13.50	70.00	3.00	2.00	1.50	10.00	330
Legumes and Nuts							
Kidney beans	24.00	55.00	2.00	2.50	4.50	12.00	330
Nuts-almonds	16.00	16.00	59.00	2.00	2.00	5.00	600
Fruits							
Apples-pears	0.50	13.00	0.25	0.25	2.00	84.00	60
Banana	0.75	18.00	0.25	0.25	0.75	80.00	80
Berries-strawberries	1.00	8.00	0.75	0.25	3.00	.87.00	40
Citrus Fruit-orange	0.75	10.00	0.25	0.50	0.50	.80.00	40
Dried Fruit-raisin	3.00	68.00	1.00	2.00	3.00	23.00	300
Grapes	0.75	17.25	0.25	0.25	0.50	81.00	75
Prunes Fruit-plums	1.00	13.00	0.25	0.25	0.50	85.00	50
Vegetables							
Brassicas-broccoli	3.50	5.00	0.25	0.25	1.00	90.00	35
Bulb Vegetables-onion	1.50	7.00	0.00	0.50	1.00	90.00	35
Fruit Vegetables-tomato	0.50	3.00	0.00	0.50	1.00	95.00	15
Mushrooms	2.00	0.00	0.25	0.25	5.50	92.00	10
Root Vegetables-carrots	1.50	8.00	0.00	0.50	1.00	89.00	20
Salad Leaves-lettuce	1.50	3.00	0.25	0.50	1.00	93.00	15
Stalk Vegetables-celery	2.25	3.00	0.25	0.50	1.00	93.00	15
Tubers-potato	2.00	17.00	0.00	0.50	0.50	80.00	80
Milk							
Cheese-cheddar	25.00	2.00	29.00	4.00	0.00	40.00	400
Cow's milk	3.00	4.50	4.00	1.00	0.00	87.00	65

Protein Group

Legumes

High in food value and fine in flavor, legumes such as peas and beans come as near as possible to being perfect vegetables. Legumes supply important quantities of protein and are low in fat (see Table 5.1). As discussed earlier in chapter 2, these can be used in combination with other foods such as cereal grains to provide a high quality protein. They are valuable in any diet and invaluable to vegetarians. There are many varieties of legumes, including lima beans, split peas, lentils, red kidney beans, pinto beans, mung beans, black-eyed peas, chickpeas and many others. Peas are the most successful of all frozen vegetables since they do not lose their vitamin C when frozen. In the process of canning, however, peas lose most of their vitamin C value. Dried beans and peas are bursting with protein--about 20 percent. It puts them on a par with meat; in fact they are better because of their low fat value as compared to meat. The same is true for the protein values of chickpeas and other legumes such as lentils. In addition to protein, legumes supply important quantities of iron, thiamin, riboflavin and trace minerals. Dried legumes lack vitamin C but by sprouting them they can be made rich in both C and B vitamins.

Nuts

Nuts are high in protein and fat, which makes them an important meat replacement for a vegetarian. The commonly used edible nuts are peanuts, almonds, walnuts, cashews, pecans, Brazil nuts, chestnuts, pistachios, filberts, hazelnuts, and macadamias. The nutritional value of different nuts varies. Most are rich in protein: almonds 20 percent, cashews 17 percent, Brazil nuts 13 percent, walnuts 12 percent. Peanuts and pine nuts are even richer in protein. Peanuts are 28 percent and pine nuts 31 percent protein. Nuts are delicious foods with natural flavors. However, you might have come across bitter almonds which are so bitter as to be inedible-- fortunately so, since they contain a harmful substance called prussic acid. Since nuts are high in fat (except chestnuts), they digest slowly and help in delaying a feeling of hunger. Nuts are a good source of B-complex vitamins, thiamin, riboflavin and niacin and of the minerals iron, copper, phosphorus and manganese. They also contain varying amounts of calcium, depending upon the variety. Walnuts, and flaxseed contain a type of fat called Omega 3. Omega-3 fatty acids are known for their positive effect on reducing Triglycerides (another type of blood fat) and for making blood less sticky and less likely to clot thus reducing the chances of heart attacks and strokes.

Fruit-Vegetable Group

Vegetables

All vegetables are good sources of minerals, vitamins and fiber. Selection of quality produce and careful adherence to proper food preparation techniques are imperative in order to get the highest food value from vegetables. Nature provides the proper foods for the proper season, so try to use freshly harvested vegetables. Many families obtain fresh vegetables from a garden planted in the back yard. The nutritive value of frozen vegetables is equal to that of fresh ones, but when vegetables are canned some nutritive elements are lost. Although many vegetables can be eaten raw, others require cooking which needs proper attention to retain the food value. As a general rule, the shorter time you cook most vegetables, the better. This does not refer to vegetables such as potatoes or squash which may be baked for a longer time if left whole in their skins. Many vitamins are water-soluble. If vegetables are boiled in a lot of water and then the water is poured down the drain, much of the nutrition goes with it. One good method to cook vegetables such as carrots or beets is to grate them, put a small amount of oil in a sauce pan, add the grated vegetable, cover, and steam for about 3 minutes over medium heat. Oil frying has the advantage of locking in the vitamins.

Vegetables may be classified according to the part of the plant used for food and according to nutritive value. Different parts of vegetables vary in nutritive value.

Green Leafy and Flowering Vegetables: Lettuce, romaine, chicory, cabbage, collards, Chinese cabbage, escarole, endive and all greens are examples of green leafy vegetables. Broccoli and cauliflower are the most commonly used flowering vegetables. Salad is one of the most popular vegetarian dishes in the West. Salad usually contains lettuce (the most popular salad plant) or a mixture of several raw green leaves. In many European countries salad is eaten with the main meal, but in the United States it is often eaten at the start of a meal. The latter has an advantage in that you are likely to eat more health-promoting salad when you are hungry at the start of a meal. Eating salad helps to avoid the danger of obesity because salad is low in calories. Also the bulkiness of salad, and the time taken to eat it, lessen intake of more fattening food. Mixed salads often contain tomatoes, cucumber, beets and scallions in addition to lettuce and various other ingredients. Try to avoid dressing or use low fat dressing or for taste lemon juice or vinegar along with a little salt and black pepper may be added.

On nutritional counts, green vegetables are most valuable in their amounts of minerals, vitamins and cellulose. They are important sources of the minerals calcium and iron and of the vitamins A, K and riboflavin, and they are valuable sources of vitamin C. The young, tender growing leaves contain more vitamin C than the mature plants. The carotene in green vegetables can be converted into vitamin A by the human body and the amount of carotene is more or less related to the amount of green pigment; therefore greener vegetables are richer in vitamin A. Among flowering vegetables, broccoli, being greener, rates higher in nutritive value than cauliflower and is a good source of iron, phosphorus, vitamin A, vitamin C and riboflavin. Cauliflower is also a good source of vitamin C; one half cup of cooked cauliflower contains about 70 milligrams of vitamin C. The leafy green and flowering vegetables are generally low in calories (Table 5.1).

Underground (Root and Tubers) Vegetables: Carrots, beets, turnips, radishes, rutabaga, kohlrabi, and parsnips are examples of root vegetables (modified roots), while potatoes, artichokes, and sweet potatoes are examples of tubers (modified underground stems). The yellow and orange varieties are rich sources of carotene. The deeper the yellow color, the greater the content of carotene, which is the precursor of vitamin A. The main virtue of most roots lies in their mineral content, but they also have value in their low-calorie bulk, so that they fill without fattening. There is also the likelihood that you will at least enjoy some of them, if not all, for their flavor. Radishes and beets, for example, are flavorful additions to green salads and contribute not more than 30 calories per hundred grams. Carrots have the additional merit of being very rich in carotene, which the body converts into vitamin A. To ensure that this substance is not squandered, the carrots should not be deep scraped or peeled for the greatest concentration of carotene is in the skin or just beneath it. Root vegetables in general are good sources of thiamin. Some have a moderate amount of vitamin C; Kohlrabi, for example, contains as much vitamin C as oranges. The underground stems or tubers, of potatoes, yams and artichokes provides a substantial amount of energy-giving starch. Sweet potatoes and artichokes have a sweeter taste than that of other tubers because they also contain some sugars. The caloric values of tubers are higher than root vegetables because of their higher carbohydrate content (see Table 5. 1). Potatoes contain ascorbic acid (vitamin C), thiamin and niacin which can add significantly to the daily allowance, if potatoes are properly prepared and consumed in sufficient quantity. The deep peeling of a potato results in a loss of up to a quarter of the potato's protein because protein is most highly concentrated just below the skin. If a peeled potato is boiled, up to half of its vitamin C content is dissolved in the cooking water. So to retain as many nutrients as possible, bake or boil unpeeled potatoes.

Stem or Stalk Vegetables: Celery and asparagus are common examples of stem vegetables. They contain minerals and vitamins in proportion to the green color, similar to that found in green leafy vegetables. Celery, being low in calories (Table 5.1) and good in taste, is most popular among people on a diet; its caloric values, in fact, are so low that digesting celery may use more energy than that provided by its nutrient contents. Asparagus contains a considerable amount of protein, a fair amount of ascorbic acid and is exceptionally rich in folic acid (member of vitamin B-complex).

Fruit Vegetables: The common examples of fruit vegetables are tomato, pepper, cucumber, squash, pumpkin, and eggplant; all of these are actually the fruit of a plant. Growing fat on fruit vegetables is unlikely because these contain more than 90 percent water, only the merest trace of fat, and very little carbohydrate. The avocado (which stands out among vegetables and fruit) is the exception and it contains 17 percent fat. Fruit vegetables have little caloric value, but our diet would be poorer without them. The fruit vegetable that exceeds all others in flavor is the tomato. Eaten raw it is a good source of carotene and vitamin C, and is low in calories; half a pound of raw tomatoes provides only 35 calories. Peppers are another exceptionally good source of vitamin C. They contain about six times as much as tomatoes. Remember, the deeper the green or yellow color, the greater the carotene (precursor of vitamin A) content of a vegetable. Another fruit vegetable, cucumber is not nutritionally important but has a unique flavor when eaten raw or cooked. Although some people dislike cucumbers because they are hard to digest, the cucumbers can be made less indigestible by thinly slicing the unpeeled cucumber, sprinkling it with salt and then after about an hour pouring off the resulting liquid.

Bulb Vegetables: Onions and garlic are the most universally used and apparently the most indispensable vegetables. Possibly they make people feel good because onions are known to improve the circulation of the blood. It has now been discovered that onions reduce serum cholesterol, thus helping to lessen the likelihood of coronary heart disease. Onions are also known to stimulate natural contractions of the intestine. Another therapeutic property of onions is to fight infections of the nose and throat, because they contain allyl aldehyde, a chemical that can kill bacteria and viruses. Nutritionally, onions are high in sulfur and a fair source of vitamin C. The old myths that onion juice rubbed on a bald head will grow hair or that onions cure boils, restore bad eyesight, reduce blood pressure, increase lust, clean out the bowels and induce sleep have not yet been substantiated by scientific evidence.

Similarly, old claims for garlic include that it made peasants work harder and soldiers fight more stubbornly. Health food literature still frequently gives the impression that garlic will cure all ills, arthritis among them. Recent scientific studies, however, have reported that garlic may help increase life span by inhibiting cholesterol accumulations, thus reducing atherosclerosis fat deposits. It has also been found that garlic helps to fight infections because of antimicrobial properties. The active ingredient, called 'allicin,' short for allyl disulfide, kills bacteria and inhibits growth of a fungus that causes meningitis, as well as fungi that cause vaginal yeast infections and athletes foot. Furthermore, garlic has been shown to reduce blood fats, blood sugars and increase blood insulin, the latter being helpful in the treatment of diabetes. Garlic as well as onions act as blood thinners and reduce the chances of blocking blood vessels. The most active blood thinning ingredient in garlic is ajoene after ajo (pronounced aho) in Spanish for garlic. (Daily dosages required for any of the benefits, however, are as high as half a head of fresh cloves.)

Mushrooms: Mushrooms do not contain chlorophyll, the green pigment found in other plants, so, instead of converting inorganic substances into organic, as green plants do, these have, like animals, to feed on organic material. There are numerous varieties of edible wild mushrooms but whoever plans to eat wild mushrooms should have a first-rate field guide to distinguish between edible and poisonous species. As a safe alternative, mass-produced cultivated mushrooms are usually available throughout the year. Besides adding flavor to many dishes, mushrooms are a good source of niacin as well as potassium and phosphorus.

Fruit

An apple a day is supposed to keep the doctor away because apples, like fruits in general, provide energy through their carbohydrate content; they add roughage to the diet; and they are a good source of natural minerals and vitamins. Fruits in general contain very little protein and are practically fat free. Two exceptions to the fat rule are avocados (also mentioned earlier under fruit vegetables) and olives, both of which contain appreciable amounts of fat. Fruits vary widely in their carbohydrate content (see Table 5.1) and have a comparatively low caloric value when fresh. Dried fruit such as raisins and fruits canned with sugar have increased calories. Although all fruits contribute some ascorbic acid, the citrus fruits are outstanding as a source of this vitamin. For example, one medium-size orange will furnish the normal adult daily requirement. Fruits also supply varying amounts of vitamin A and the B-complex vitamins. The yellow fruits, such as peaches, cantaloupe and apricots are good sources of the pigment carotene, a precursor of vitamin A. Plums and dried fruits are the best sources of thiamin. Fruits in general contribute appreciable amounts of the minerals iron and calcium. Among the fruits richest in iron are dried fruits of all kinds (raisins, dates, dried figs, prunes) as well as apricots, peaches, bananas, grapes and berries. Calcium is found in citrus fruits, strawberries and dried figs. Dried figs are also high in fiber and protein as well as in B vitamins; their gentle laxative action adds to their health-giving properties. Sodium, magnesium and potassium are present in varying amounts in most fruits.

Careful preparation and storage of fruits is essential to retain the maximum value of vitamins and minerals. For example, clinical studies reveal that many children and adults do not get enough ascorbic acid even though the consumption of citrus fruits has increased greatly in the last century; this is due to lack of knowledge about its sources, preparation and storage, rather than to cost or availability. If peeling is required, for instance, fruit should be peeled thinly to conserve the nutrients. Fresh fruit should be chilled before the juice is extracted, which should be done just before serving. This is because bruising, cutting, and allowing fruit juice to be exposed to the air causes considerable loss of ascorbic acid. If juices are stored in a refrigerator, they should be put in covered containers (preferably air tight) to reduce oxidation and loss of vitamin C. The fruits which can be frozen compare favorably to fresh ones in nutritive value.

Milk Group

A breast-fed infant and a suckled calf are both getting their perfect food--mother's milk which is nature's way to perfect nutrition. Although the milk of all mammals has the same constituents, the proportion of constituents differs. For example, human milk contains less protein and more carbohydrate than cow's milk (Table 5.2). By any standard, milk is still the most valuable of any food in the human diet; it contains high-quality protein (mainly casein with small amounts of lactalbumin and lactoglobulin), fat (cream), carbohydrate (lactose or milk sugar), the minerals calcium and phosphorus, and the vitamins riboflavin, niacin, vitamin A and (when the milk is fortified) vitamin D (see Table 5.2). The exact composition of milk varies to some degree with the breed of cattle, the season of the year, and the feed given to the animal.

Table 5.2. Nutrient content of cow's milk, human milk, and infant formula per liter.

Nutrient	Cows milk	Human milk	Typical Infant Formula
Calories	670	750	680
Protein (g) (Casein, Lactalbumin)	36	11	16
Carbohydrate (g) (Lactose)	49	68	72
Fat (g)	36	45	36
Cholesterol (mg)	113	200	160
Vitamin A (I.U.)	1,447	1,898	2,500
Vitamin D (l.U.)	400	22	400
Vitamin E (I.U.)	1.5	2.7	15
Vitamin C (I.U.)	10	43	55
Folacin (microgram)	55	52	50

Niacin (milligram equiv.)	9.5	1.5	7.0
Riboflavin (mg)	1.8	0.36	1.0
Thian-in (mg)	0.3	0.16	0.6
Vitamin B6 (mg)	0.5	0.1	0.4
Vitamin B12 (mg)	5.3	0.3	1.5
Vitamin K (microgram)	60	15	65
Calcium (mg)	1,220	340	510
Phosphorus (mg)	960	140	390
Iodine (microgram)	47	30	68
Iron (mg)	0.5	0.2	1.5
Magnesium (mg)	120	40	41
Zinc (mg)	4	1.6	5
Copper (microgram)	300	240	400
Sodium (milliequivalents)	22	7	10
Potassium (milliequivalents)	38	13	18
Chloride (milliequivalents)	28	1.1	15

SOURCES: Fomon, *S.J. Infant Nutrition,* W.B. Saunders Co., Philadelphia, 1974. Composition of infant formulas from Ross Laboratories, Columbus, Ohio. National Dairy Council, *Newer Knowledge of Milk,* 3rd ed. Chicago, 1972.

Three-fourths of the calcium, nearly one-half of the riboflavin, and one-fourth of the protein, normally, come from milk in the average food supply. To keep calories and fat level down, the use of skim or low-fat milk is quite effective. One pint of skim milk has 180 calories as compared to one pint of whole milk which provides 320 calories. Although milk is extremely important as a rich source of protein, minerals, and vitamins for a growing child, it is still necessary for adults and senior citizens as a source of calcium. Calcium in milk appears to be extremely important in delaying deossification or osteoporosis, a bone loss which results in weakening of skeletal strength, and the occurrence of fractures with just minimal stress. If milk is not liked as a beverage, it can be taken in the form of cheese or yogurt or used in various other dishes involving milk or milk products.

To make milk safe from any kind of pathogenic bacteria, most milk is pasteurized, even though this process destroys some of the thiamin and vitamin C. The pasteurization of milk involves heating milk to destroy pathogenic bacteria and then cooling it rapidly. If milk is not pasteurized, a home pasteurization (heating of milk until it comes to a boil) is generally useful. Certified milk is not pasteurized but must meet standards of cleanliness. Milk may also be homogenized, a process that reduces the size of the cream particles. As a result, the cream does not rise to the top of the milk but stays suspended throughout the liquid.

Cheese: Milk or cheese is one of the meat alternatives because of the similarity of nutrients, particularly animal proteins. The nutrients in cheese are more concentrated than in milk (Table 5.1), and cheese is an excellent source of protein and also of calcium, riboflavin and vitamin A. But with the exception of such low-fat cheeses as cottage cheese, it is also high in saturated fat and cholesterol. Thus, moderate consumption of cheese is wise, especially for those with heart problems. The type of milk used in the manufacture of cheese reflects the nutritive qualities of the cheese. For example, protein, calcium, and vitamin B factors are contributed by the whole milk used in cheddar cheese--often called American cheese. Cottage cheese (unripened soft cheese) is less concentrated than cheddar cheese, with about four-fifths as much protein per pound.

Yogurt: Of all dairy foods, health food lovers rank yogurt as supreme. Yogurt is one of the oldest health foods. The ancient Hebrews ate yogurt, as did the Egyptians. In the book of Genesis there is a mention that Abraham ate yogurt and served it to his guests. Yogurt is a staple of the Bulgarians, who eat it daily and have one of the highest rates of longevity in the world. Yogurt is one food that has long been associated with the attainment of great age. Yogurt contains more protein and riboflavin than milk itself and is more easily digested.

Yogurt is a fermented milk product made from whole, low-fat or skim milk. The bacteria usually used are *Lactobacillus bulgaricus, Streptococcus thermophilus* and possibly *Lactobacillus acidophilus.* Yogurt retains all the food value of the milk from which it is made. Yogurt is not exceptionally low in calories unless it is made from skim milk and is unsweetened.

Table 5.3. Summary of Vegetarian Foods that Heal

Food	Healing Value				
Apples	Protects your heart	prevents constipation	Blocks diarrhea	Improves lung capacity	Cushions joints
Apricots	Combats cancer	Controls blood pressure	Saves your eyesight	Sheilds against Alzheimer's	Slows aging process
Artichokes	Aids digestion	Lowers cholesterol	Protects your heart	Stabilizes blood sugar	Guards against liver disease
Avocadoes	Battles diabetes	Lowers cholesterol	Helps stops strokes	Controls blood pressure	Smoothes skin
Bananas	Protects your heart	Quiets a cough	Strengthens bones	Controls blood pressure	Blocks diarrhea
Beans	Prevents constipation	Helps hemorroids	Lowers cholesterol	Combats cancer	Stabilizes blood sugar
Beets	Controls blood pressure	Combats cancer	Strengthens bones	Protects your heart	Aids weight loss
Blueberries	Combats cancer	Protects your heart	Stabilizes blood sugar	Boosts memory	Prevents constipation
Broccoli	Strengthens bones	Saves eyesight	Combats cancer	Protects your heart	Controls blood pressure
Cabbage	Combats cancer	Prevents constipation	Promotes weight loss	Protects your heart	Helps hemorroids
Canteloupe	Saves eyesight	Controls blood pressure	Lowers cholesterol	Combats cancer	Supports immune system
Carrots	Saves eyesight	Protects your heart	Prevents constipation	Combats cancer	Promotes wt loss

Cauliflower	Protects against Prostate Cancer	Combats Breast Cancer	Strengthens bones	Banishes bruises	Guards against heart disease
Cherries	Protects your heart	Combats Cancer	Ends insomnia	Slows aging process	Sheilds against Alzheimer's
Chestnuts	Promotes weight loss	Protects your heart	Lowers cholesterol	Combats Cancer	Controls blood pressure
[Chili] Peppers	Aids digestion	Soothes sore throat	Clears sinuses	Combats Cancer	Boosts immune system
Figs	Promotes weight loss	Helps stops strokes	Lowers cholesterol	Combats Cancer	Controls blood pressure
Flax	Aids digestion	Battles diabetes	Protects your heart	Improves mental health	Boosts immune system
Garlic	Lowers cholesterol	Controls blood pressure	Combats cancer	kills bacteria	Fights fungus
Grapefruit	Protects against heart attacks	Promotes Weight loss	Helps stops strokes	Combats Prostate Cancer	Lowers cholesterol
Grapes	saves eyesight	Conquers kidney stones	Combats cancer	Enhances blood flow	Protects your heart
Green tea	Combats cancer	Protects your heart	Helps stops strokes	Promotes Weight loss	Kills bacteria
Honey	Heals wounds	Aids digestion	Guards against ulcers	Increases energy	Fights allergies
Lemons	Combats cancer	Protects your heart	Controls blood pressure	Smoothes skin	Stops scurvy
Limes	Combats cancer	Protects your heart	Controls blood pressure	Smoothes skin	Stops scurvy
Mangoes	Combats cancer	Boosts memory	Regulates thyroid	aids digestion	Sheilds against Alzheimer's
Mushrooms	Controls blood pressure	Lowers cholesterol	Kills bacteria	Combats cancer	Strengthens bones
Oats	Lowers cholesterol	Combats cancer	Battles diabetes	prevents constipation	Smoothes skin
Olive oil	Protects your heart	Promotes Weight loss	Combats cancer	Battles diabetes	Smoothes skin
Onions	Reduce risk of heart attack	Combats cancer	Kills bacteria	Lowers cholesterol	Fights fungus
Oranges	Supports immune systems	Combats cancer	Protects your heart	Stregthens respiration	
Peaches	prevents constipation	Combats cancer	Helps stops strokes	aids digestion	Helps hemorroids
Peanuts	Protects against heart disease	Promotes Weight loss	Combats Prostate Cancer	Lowers cholesterol	Aggravates diverticulitis
Pineapple	Strengthens bones	Relieves colds	Aids digestion	Dissolves warts	Blocks diarrhea

Prunes	Slows aging process	prevents constipation	boosts memory	Lowers cholesterol	Protects against heart disease
Rice	Protects your heart	Battles diabetes	Conquers kidney stones	Combats cancer	Helps stops strokes
Strawberries	Combats cancer	Protects your heart	boosts memory	Calms stress	
Sweet Potatoes	Saves your eyesight	Lifts mood	Combats cancer	Strengthens bones	
Tomatoes	Protects prostate	Combats cancer	Lowers cholesterol	Protects your heart	
Walnuts	Lowers cholesterol	Combats cancer	boosts memory	Lifts mood	Protects against heart disease
Water	Promotes Weight loss	Combats cancer	Conquers kidney stones	Smooths skin	
Watermelon	Protects prostate	Promotes Weight loss	Lowers cholesterol	Helps stops strokes	Controls blood pressure
Wheat germ	Combats Colon Cancer	prevents constipation	Lowers cholesterol	Helps stops strokes	improves digestion
Wheat bran	Combats Colon Cancer	prevents constipation	Lowers cholesterol	Helps stops strokes	improves digestion
Yogurt	Guards against ulcers	Strengthens bones	Lowers cholesterol	Supports immune systems	Aids digestion

Chapter 6

VEGETABLE THAT HEALS:
Health Benefits of Okra *(Hibiscus esculentus)*

Health benefits of Okra
Okra Recipes
Okra Gardening Experience
How to Freeze Okra
Seed Source

Health Benefits of Okra *(Hibiscus esculentus)*

A guy had been suffering from constipation for the past 20 years and recently from acid reflux. He didn't realize that the treatment could be so simple -- OKRA! He started eating okra within the last 2 months and since then have never taken medication again. All he did was eat 6 pieces of OKRA everyday. He's now regular and his blood sugar has dropped from 135 to 98, with his cholesterol and acid reflux also under control. Here are some facts on okra (from the research of Ms. Sylvia Zook, PH.D (nutrition), University of Illinois.

"Okra is a powerhouse of valuable nutrients, nearly half of which is soluble fiber in the form of gums and pectins. Soluble fiber helps to lower serum cholesterol, reducing the risk of heart disease. The other half is insoluble fiber which helps to keep the intestinal tract healthy, decreasing the risk of some forms of cancer, especially colo-rectal cancer. Nearly 10% of the recommended levels of vitamin B6 and folic acid is also present in a half cup of cooked okra.

Okra is a rich source of many nutrients, including fiber, vitamin B6 and folic acid. Here're the following numbers from the University of Illinois Extension Okra Page. [Please check there for more details.]

Okra Nutrition (half-cup cooked okra)
* Calories = 25
* Dietary Fiber = 2 grams
* Protein = 1.5 grams
* Carbohydrates = 5.8 grams
* Vitamin A = 460 IU
* Vitamin C = 13 mg
* Folic acid = 36.5 micrograms
* Calcium = 50 mg
* Iron = 0.4 mg
* Potassium = 256 mg
* Magnesium = 46 mg

These numbers should be used as a guideline only, and if you are on a medically-restricted diet please consult your physician and/or dietician.

Ms Sylvia W. Zook, Ph.D. (nutritionist) has very kindly provided the following thought-provoking comments on the many benefits of this versatile vegetable. They are well worth reading.

1. The superior fiber found in okra helps to stabilize blood sugar as it curbs the rate at which sugar is absorbed from the intestinal tract.

2. Okra's mucilage not only binds cholesterol but bile acid carrying toxins dumped into it by the filtering liver. But it doesn't stop there...

3. Many alternative health practitioners believe all disease begins in The colon. The okra fiber, absorbing water and ensuring bulk in stools, helps prevent constipation. Fiber in general is helpful for this but okra is one of the best, along with ground flax seed and psyllium. Unlike harsh wheat bran, which can irritate or injure the intestinal tract, okra's mucilage soothes, and okra facilitates elimination more comfortably by its slippery characteristic many people abhor. In other words, this incredibly valuable vegetable not only binds excess cholesterol and toxins (in bile acids) which cause numerous health

problems, if not evacuated, but also assures their easy passage from the body.

4. Further contributing to the health of the intestinal tract, okra fiber (as well as flax and psyllium) has no equal among fibers for feeding the good bacteria (probiotics).

5. To retain most of okra's nutrients and self-digesting enzymes , it should be cooked as little as possible, e.g. with low heat or lightly steamed. Some eat it raw.

Cholesterol lowering effects of OKRA

Okra, a fruit high in water-soluble fiber (WSF) and widely consumed in Africa was investigated as a potential candidate to decrease cholesterol. The water-soluble fiber of some fruits and vegetables has been the focus of scientific research in relation to potential health benefits to cardiovascular diseases (CVD). The 3 weeks randomized crossover placebo study carried out among 30 healthy subjects concluded that Okra is an effective cholesterol lowering dietary adjunct. Okra might therefore be an interesting approach in the prevention of CVD risk factors as well as an opportunity for okra commercial challenge.

Source: Bangana, A., N. Dossou, et al. (2005). "Cholesterol lowering effects of Okra (Hibiscus esculentus) in Senegalese adult men." Annals of Nutrition and metabolism 18 (Suppl. 1): 199

Okra Against Heart Disease

For a triple-powered punch against heart disease, eat some okra. It strikes first with an antioxidant job to atherosclerosis – that dangerous hardening and clogging of your blood vessels. The top antioxidant in okra's arsenal is vitamin C which the World Health Organization has linked to a reduced risk of fatal heart disease. One cup of sliced okra has more vitamin C than a whole tomato.

Although you cannot rely on okra as a single source of this important vitamin, it makes an interesting and nutritious addition to your diet.

With a healthy dose of folate – about 40 percent of your daily requirement in each cup – okra then gives heart disease a left hook. Without this B vitamin, your body leaves behind loose amino acids, called homocysteine, when it metabolizes protein. Too much homocysteine built up in your blood damages your arteries and can lead to heart disease and stroke.

Okra gives a final knockout blow with its wealth of minerals – mainly potassium and magnesium. For lowering blood pressure, experts say eating potassium-rich foods may be as important as losing weight and cutting back on salt. And just the right amount of magnesium is especially important to seniors, who may not absorb it as well as they used to and may excrete more of it as waste. Magnesium helps control cholesterol and blood pressure, regulates your heart rhythm, and may even improve your odds of surviving heart disease and heart attacks.

Arms Against Osteoporosis

Do not forget okra when you're planning a bone-building menu. It's full of four osteoporosis-fighting nutrients – potassium, magnesium, vitamin C, and beta carotene. People who eat foods high in these nutrients, according to research from the United Kingdom, may slow down the bone loss that can lead to osteoporosis. To top it off, a cup of okra gives you over 10 percent of the recommended dietary allowance (RDA) of the most famous bone-building mineral of all – calcium.

Eases Osteoarthritis

Some doctors used to think osteoarthritis (OA), the most common type of joint disease, was unstoppable, but now natural alternatives give new hope. Foods like okra contain both vitamin C and manganese, nutrients your body needs to build up joints and cartilage. Experts who looked at a variety of research suggest a diet high in vitamin C may slow down the development of OA. They also remind us that manganese is a necessary component of cartilage

Cooking Tips and Recipes

Even though okra has a sticky reputation, do not judge this little vegetable until you have enjoyed it cooked properly. The chemical compounds that make okra gummy stay safely trapped inside each pod, unless you slice them. Steam whole pods or add them to stews for extra flavor. If you're making a gumbo, cut up the pod and let the natural juices thicken your dish. For a different taste, slice okra raw into a salad or coat the little wagon wheels with cornmeal and fry them up crisp.

HOWEVER, IF YOU ARE GOING TO FRY IT (AND IT IS UNDENIABLY DELICIOUS PREPARED THAT WAY WHEN ROLLED IN CORNMEAL AND SALT), ONLY EXTRA VIRGIN OLIVE OIL IS RECOMMENDED (THIS IS NOT THE UNHEALTHY PARTIALLY HYDROGENATED PRODUCT FOUND IN PROCESSED FOODS OR LARD USED BY RESTAURANTS.).

For best cooking results, okra should be fresh. The pods should be small (3 inches or so long), or the okra becomes tough and stringy. If choose to use frozen okra, remove as much of the moisture as possible before cooking by spreading on a paper towel, or patting it dry after it thaws.

No matter how you eat your okra, remember two things. Rub off the outer fuzz with a towel if you do not like the roughness. Avoid cooking okra in pans made of brass, iron or copper, the pods will darken.

*****

Creole Okra

Okra soaks up the flavors of tomatoes, garlic, and herbs in this tantalizing dish. You may use frozen okra if fresh is unavailable.

1 tsp. olive oil
1/2 small onion, diced
1 garlic clove, minced
1/2 small green pepper, diced
1 ripe tomato, seeded and coarsely chopped
1/2 lb. fresh okra, sliced into 1/2-inch pieces
1 tsp. dried oregano
1/2 tsp. dried thyme
Salt and freshly ground black pepper, to taste
Pinch of cayenne pepper, if desired

In a medium skillet, heat oil over medium-high heat. Add onion and
garlic and sauté 3 minutes, stirring frequently.

Add green pepper and sauté 3 to 4 minutes.

Add tomatoes and okra. Cover and cook over low heat 10 to 15 minutes, until okra is soft. Add oregano, thyme, salt and black pepper, to taste, and cayenne pepper, if using. Cook uncovered about 1 minute.

Courtesy of the American Institute for Cancer Research

*****

Okra with Potatoes

This is a delicious simple North Indian recipe. You can leave out the hot pepper if you wish.

1 (one) pound fresh Okra
One large, or two medium onions
1 (one) potato, peeled
6 tablespoons cooking oil
1 hot green pepper (remove stem, slit lengthwise)
1/2 (half) teaspoon salt
1/2 (half) teaspoon turmeric powder

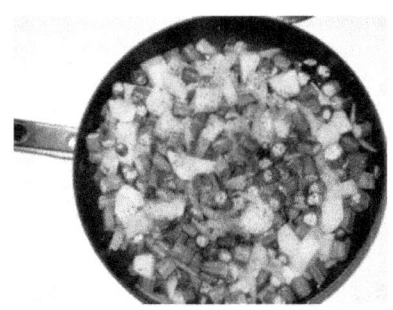

Wash okra, remove stems, cut lengthwise (about 4 pieces for each pod), then dry thoroughly on paper towels.

Slice onion thinly then separate into long pieces. Cut potatoes into cubes, about 1/2" (half inch) on side.

In large frying pan, heat oil on medium heat. Add onions and potatoes and stir until lightly browned. Add salt, turmeric and then the Okra pieces, plus the hot pepper. Cook uncovered. Stir occasionally until done (approx. 20 minutes). Serves four.

*****

Whole Okra with Onions

This is another popular North Indian okra recipe. It is better to use fresh okra (not frozen), and must not be overgrown. This is best as a side dish, probably better with breads than with rice.

1 (one) pound fresh Okra
1 (one) medium to large onion
1/2 (half) teaspoon cumin seeds
1/4 (one-fourth) teaspoon turmeric powder
1/2 (half) teaspoon mango powder [if available]
1/2 (half) teaspoon ground red pepper (optional)
1 (one) clove garlic
1/2 (half) inch piece fresh ginger
4 (four) tablespoons cooking oil
1/2 (half) teaspoon salt (or to taste)

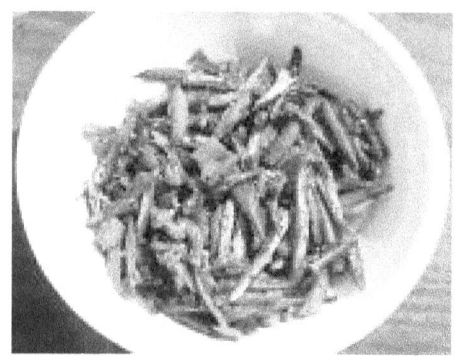

Wash okra, let dry thoroughly, or pat dry with paper towels. Remove stems, slit lengthwise once or twice (do not cut through, each pod must remain as one piece).

Chop ginger and garlic into small pieces. Slice (do not chop) the onion and separate into long strips or rings.

On medium heat, place 2 tablespoons oil in medium size non-stick pan or frying pan. Add cumin seeds. After approx. 30 seconds add garlic and ginger. When garlic is slightly browned (less than a minute) add onions. Cook for about 5 minutes until onions are lightly browned. Stir occasionally, do not overcook.

Add turmeric, pepper and mango powder, and stir to mix well. Remove onion/spice mixture from pan and save in a small bowl or plate.

In the same pan as above, add 2 tablespoons oil and okra and salt. Cook on medium heat for about 5 minutes, stirring frequently.

Lower heat slightly, cover the pan, and let cook for about 10 more minutes. Remove lid, stir and cook for another 5 to 10 minutes, until moisture is gone and okra is tender. Do not overcook, the okra should remain separate and not become mushy.

Finally, add the onion/spice mixture back with the okra, stir and serve while still warm. Serves four.

*****

Okra Casserole

Take a medium size casserole dish, spray with pam spray. Layer a layer of fresh or frozen okra, add in order, layer of chopped onion, chopped bell pepper, can of relleno tomatoes with green chilies, cheddar cheese, layer of okra, layer of onion, layer of green pepper, can of stewed tomatoes, monterey jack grated cheese, [stuff 4 slices of bacon around edges of dish to season, but leave out if you're vegetarian] salt and pepper.

Preheat oven to 375 degs. (F). Bake for 45 to 60 minutes, or until the pepper and onion are tender.

Only make one layer if you have a small family. The two layers work fine for a larger dish to take to family and gatherings. You can make this hotter by adding a little Tabasco. It is delicious.

Note: This recipe is provided by Maragret Webb of Crossville, Tennessee.

*****

Grandma's Fried Okra and Potatoes

This is a dish for those who profess to hate okra! Not the deep-fried, batter-dipped variety, this is quick -- something you can keep an eye on while the rest of your supper cooks. And remember, the larger the okra pod, the tougher, so choose small pods.

1 pound fresh okra
2 large potatoes (baking type -- not new potatoes)
1 medium white onion, finely chopped
1/2 cup cornmeal
1 teaspoon salt
1/2 cup vegetable oil
1/4 teaspoon ground pepper

Wash okra and cut off stem ends. Cut in 1/2-inch pieces. Peel potatoes and chop into 1/2-inch dice. Put okra and potatoes in large bowl. Add chopped onion to mixture. Sprinkle cornmeal, salt and pepper over mixture. Stir until cornmeal is evenly distributed throughout mixture.

Heat cooking oil in large skillet over medium heat (oil should be hot, but not smoking hot). Carefully spoon okra/potato mixture into hot oil. Fry, turning mixture occasionally, until potatoes are done and mixture is nicely browned, about 10 to 12 minutes. Drain on paper towels. Makes enough for 4 or 5 hungry people.

*****

Arkansas Fried Okra

10-12 okra, sliced
2 med. potatoes, cubed
1 med. onion, chopped
1 t. salt
pepper to taste
3 T. YELLOW corn meal
1 T. flour
6 T. margarine

Sprinkle okra with salt, pepper, corn meal, and flour. Stir until well coated. Add onions and potatoes. Do not stir. In a cast iron skillet, melt margarine on medium heat. Add vegetables. Cook until tender and coating becomes crusty and well browned. Stir at intervals. Serve hot and eat it all because it is not good warmed over.

*****

Grilled Okra

15 to 20 tender okra pods, 3 inches long
Olive Oil
Cajun Seasoning

Place okra on a metal or wooden skewer through the side at the center of the pod. Brush with Olive Oil. Sprinkle on Cajun Seasoning.

Grill on charcoal or gas grill for 2 to 3 minutes then turn over and grill until turning brown.

Serve and eat while still warm.

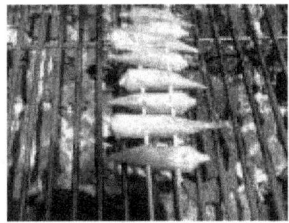

Note: Using 2 skewers and building like a ladder works a lot better than trying to turn the okra on just 1 skewer. Make an individual ladder for each guest. (see picture above)
Provided by Travis Hall from Belton, Texas.

*****
Texas Fried Okra

    1 pound okra
    cornmeal
    Virgin Olive Oil [replace "lard" for a healthy recipe]
    salt and pepper

Wash okra, cut off stems and cut diagonally into 1/4 inch slices. Sprinkle with salt and pepper, then dredge in cornmeal, tossing and turning the okra in the meal until thoroughly coated. Heat olive oil in a heavy skillet, the size depending on the quantity of okra. Add okra and fry over moderate heat. When the pieces on the bottom are brown, turn with a spatula so the rest can brown evenly. When done, skim out with perforated spatula. Drain on paper before serving.

Serving Size : 4
[Note: Provided from "The Wide, Wide World of Texas Cooking"]

*****

Smothered Okra and Tomatoes

2 pounds okra
3 tablespoons oil
1 tablespoon all-purpose flour
1 onion, chopped
1/2 bell pepper, chopped
2 ribs celery, chopped
5 tomatoes, chopped
Creole Seasoning*

Wash okra. Cut in 1/8 inch slices. Fry in an aluminum pot on medium heat in 2 tablespoons oil until okra is no longer sticky.

In another skillet, make a medium dark roux with 1 tablespoon oil and flour. Add onion, bell pepper, and celery. Simmer until tender. Add tomatoes and simmer for 5 minutes. Add okra, seasoned with Creole Seasoning.

Simmer for 1 hour.

Yields 6 servings.

* Creole seasoning:

2 Tbs ground cayenne
2 Tbs black pepper
4 Tbs paprika
1 tsp dried thyme
1 tsp dried oregano
1/2 Tbs garlic powder
1 tsp onion powder

Place in jar and shake.

Cheaper than the prepared stuff if you already have the spices.

*****

Gumbo recipe

You can follow this fantastic recipe in a slow cooker with no oil.

1 onion chopped
3 cloves (that's cloves not cloves of garlic)
1 green pepper, diced
2 cups diced tomatoes
4 cups vegetable stock
1 cup cooked lima beans (also known as butter beans)
1 cup fresh (or frozen) corn
1.5 cups sliced okra
1 tsp salt
1/4 tsp allspice

Sauté the onion and green pepper with the cloves in water until soft. Remove the cloves. Put all ingredients in a slow cooker on high for 6 hours or low for 8-10 hours.
Pretty simple! It's nice to come home at the end of the day and have everything ready.

*****

Syrian-Style Okra with Dried Fruit

1/2 pound okra, chopped
1/2 small onion, peeled and finely chopped
1 tsp. oil
1 tbsp. water
1 1/2 cup dried fruit (about 8 oz. prunes, apricots, raisins, etc.)
1/2 cup prune juice
1/2 cup tomato juice
1/4 lemon, minced (rind and fruit)

Stir-fry okra and onion with oil and water in a large frying pan for 5 minutes over medium heat. Add dried fruit, juices, and lemon.

Simmer 15 minutes, stirring often. Serve warm or chilled. Serves 4.

Calories per serving, 267; fat, 1 gram; carbohydrates, 68 grams.

*****

Bamia Ladyfinger Relish
(Island of Zanzibar)

"Ladyfingers" is the African/British name for okra and a fitting one for a delicate vegetable that we do not use nearly enough. Of course, the relish is best if made with fresh okra. Frozen (or even canned) okra is a compromise but it does make a new and different relish to add to your menu.

    2 Tbs. Oil
    1/2 cup chopped Onions
    2 cloves Garlic
    Chili Pepper (or use 1 tsp. crushed red pepper)
    1 inch Fresh Ginger (or use 1 tsp. ground ginger).
    2 pound Fresh OKRA, trimmed at ends and cut in 1 inch slices
    (or drain two 16 oz. cans of okra).

In an electric skillet or large frying pan Sauté: 1/2 cup Onion in 2 Tbs. Oil until slightly brown.
    Add to oil other ingredients and sauté for 1 minute.
    Add 2 pound Fresh OKRA, trimmed at ends and cut in 1 inch slices (or drain two 16 oz. cans of okra). Sauté for several minutes.

Add fresh tomato cut in thin strips. Sauté for 5 minutes.

Pack into hot sterile jar. Yield: 1 quart

Serve hot or cold as a side relish dish with other dishes including meats and fish.

*****

Smothered Okra, Eggplant and Tomato

SEASONING MIX
1 1/2 teaspoons onion powder
1 teaspoon salt (omit if use canned tomatoes with salt)
1 teaspoon dried mustard
1 teaspoon dried thyme leaves
1/2 teaspoon garlic powder
1/2 teaspoon ground black pepper
1/2 teaspoon ground white pepper (or use all black)
1/2 teaspoon dill weed
1/8 teaspoon cayenne pepper (red pepper)
****

2 cups chopped onion, in all
1 cup chopped green bell pepper (or red bell pepper)
2 cups chopped okra, in all
1 medium eggplant, peeled --- 1 cup finely diced, remaining medium diced.
3 cups fresh tomatoes chopped, or 2 cans diced tomatoes
1/2 cup tomato sauce (omit if using canned tomatoes which already have lots of juice)
1 cup apple juice

1. Mix seasoning spices in a small bowl.

2. Combine 1 cup of chopped onion, 1 cup finely chopped eggplant, 1 cup of okra (you can put in a food processor and pulse to chop finely)

3. Heat non-stick skillet or pot over high heat about 4 minutes. Add chopped vegetables, bell pepper and seasoning mix, stir and cook for about 5 minutes. Vegetables should stick to bottom of pan, then you unstick and stir them so that they caramelize (brown) a little but don't burn.

4. Stir in 1 cup of apple juice, stir to unstick from bottom, add 1 cup of tomatoes. Cook, stirring occasionally until most of liquid evaporates, about 20 minutes.

5. Add remaining onions, okra, eggplant and tomatoes (tomato sauce if used). Scrape to clear bottom and cook 10 minutes or more until eggplant is cooked.

Notes: In Oklahoma in the heat of August Okra is about the only vegetable that still grows (even the tomatoes stop setting fruit when it gets too hot). You can also use frozen okra. When well cooked, the gumminess goes away and its serves as a thickener to the dish. If you're wary of okra, you might want to reduce the total amount to 1 cup and let the eggplant and tomatoes dominate. You can use onion powder and garlic powder in the spice mixes, which is redundant when using real onions, but it actually imparts a different flavor. cooking the vegetables a long time in a non-stick skillet and letting them brown a little to caramelize and develop the flavors is worth, and pays to be patient.

*****

Just Okra

    1/2 Pound Okra
    Salt to taste.
    1 Tsp (or to taste) Paprika or Chili Powder
    1/2 Tsp.Turmeric
    2 Tsp. Oil
    1 Tbsp. Plain Yogurt
    1 Tsp. Mustard Seeds

Wash and Cut the Okra into round pieces.

Heat oil in a pan add in Mustard seeds. Add okra and Stir. Mix spices and cover. Cook on low flame.
Add Yogurt and stir. Cook till it is dry.
Enjoy as a side dish.

NOTE: Okra has a tendency to stick the pan. Adding Yogurt prevents it from sticking, gives a tart flavor and helps maintain the green color.

*****

Okra Yogurt Salad

10 Okra cut into small rounds
1 Cup Plain Yoghurt
Salt to taste.
1 Tsp Oil
1 Tsp Paprika or to taste.
1 Tsp Mustard seeds (optional).

Wash and cut the Okra. Beat Yoghurt thick and add salt.

Heat a pan with oil, add mustard seeds and Okra. Cover & let cook a couple of minutes. Add Paprika and stir.

Cool and add to Yoghurt , Chill & serve .

Okra is also referred as lady's finger in English & Bhindi in Hindi

*****

Okra Pickles

Pickled Okra

White vinegar (heated to boiling and poured over okra packed in jars)
Garlic (about a teaspoon finely chopped, fresh or bought in jars)
Dill Seed (2 pinches)
Dill Weed (fresh or dry, 2 pinches)
Red Pepper Flakes (a sprinkle or two, your taste)
Alum (a dash)
Salt (a dash)
Sweetener (of your choice, to cut the bite of the vinegar, a pinch)

Note: Provided by Mike Warren of San Antonio, Texas

*****

Dill Pickled Okra

2 pounds young okra
celery leaves
4 cloves
4 sprigs dill
2 cups water
2 cups white vinegar
4 tsp salt

1. Scrub okra and pack whole pods into clean, hot jars. In each jar insert a few celery leaves, 1 garlic clove, peeled, and 1 sprig of dill.

2. Bring water, vinegar, and salt to a boil. Pour the boiling liquid over the okra.

3. Seal and process 10 minutes in simmering hot water.

4. Let okra stand for about 1 month before using.

Makes 4 pints.

NOTE: RECIPE FROM THE UNIVERSITY OF CALIFORNIA COOPERATIVE EXTENSION IN LOS ANGELES COUNTY.

*****

Okra Pickles

Lady Bird Johnson's version of a traditional Texas pickle.

3 Lbs. Okra
6 Hot Peppers
6 Cloves Garlic - Peeled
1 Qt. Distilled Vinegar
1-1/3 Cups Water
1/2 Cup Salt
1 Tbsp Mustard Seed

Clean okra and pack in clean canning jars.

Place one pepper and one garlic clove in each jar.

Combine remaining ingredients in stainless steel or other corrosion resistant pot and bring to a full boil. Pour over packed okra to 1/2 inch from top of jars. Cover jars with new canning lids.

Process in boiling water for ten minutes.

Eating tip: When eating okra pickles if you are going to take a bite out one rather than putting the whole thing in your mouth, bite the tip rather than the stem end. This avoids possible issues of spray

*****

Pickled Okra
 (BY CHUCK TAGGART)

> 5 pounds okra
> 8 cups vinegar
> 1 cup water
> 1/2 cup kosher salt
> 8 cloves garlic
> 8 or more dried or fresh chilies (pepper)

Wash okra, leaving top cam and removing excess stem. Combine vinegar, water and kosher salt. Bring to a boil. Drop okra into boiling mixture (and chilies if you're using fresh chilies) and bring to a rolling boil. Place in hot, pint-sized sterilized jars. Add one clove of garlic and, if you're using dried instead of fresh chilies, one or more dried hot chilies (depending on how hot you want them) to each jar. Seal while hot. Let stand 8 - 10 weeks before serving.

*****

Spicy Pickled Okra

> 3 pounds okra, whole
> 6 hot red or green peppers

6 garlic cloves
1 quart vinegar, 5% acidity
1 1/3 cups water
1/2 cup salt
1 tbsp mustard seeds

Wash okra. Trim stems; do not cut into pods. Pack okra into clean, hot pint jars; add hot pepper and garlic clove to each jar.

Bring remaining ingredients to a boil. Cover okra with hot liquid, filling to 1/2 inch from top. Adjust jar lids.

Process 10 minutes in boiling water. (Start to count processing time as soon as water in canner returns to boiling.) Remove jars.

Set jars upright on a wire rack or folded towel to cool. Place them several inches apart. Yield: 6 pints.

*****

Pickled Okra
(from Vegetarian Resource Center - Boston, USA)

1 pound tender young okra
1/2 small habanera or other hot chile, sliced thin, or to taste
1 small onion, sliced thin
2 cloves garlic, sliced thin
1 cup water
3 cups distilled white vinegar
1 tablespoon pickling spice
2 tablespoons salt (optional)

Wash the okra and pick it over, removing any pods that are hard and woody and any with soft spots.

Pack the okra into hot sterilized pint canning jars, stem ends down. Place the remaining ingredients into a nonreactive saucepan and bring them to a boil over medium heat.

Remove from the heat and slowly pout over the okra in the jars. Seal the jars according to proper canning procedures, and store them in a cool dark place for 4 weeks, then serve as a condiment.
Makes about 2 pints.

*****

Pickled Okra
(BY CHEF RICK)

2 pounds fresh okra
5 cloves garlic, peeled
1 quart white vinegar
1/2 cup water
8 tablespoons pickling salt
1 tablespoon celery seed

Wash okra. Using manufacturer's directions, sterilize five one-pint jars along with lids and rings.

Pack okra in jars, alternating facing up and down until jars are full. Mix remaining ingredients and bring to a boil. Pour over okra and seal. Let stand 3 weeks before serving. Chill before serving for added crispness.

*****

Okra Gardening Experiences

Okra grows in warmer climate. You will not have luck to grow in places like Colorado Springs, Colorado at 7,000 feet or so. However, you may be able to grow in greenhouse anywhere. The personal accounts from various places will give you good idea about growing Okra and kind of climate it needs.

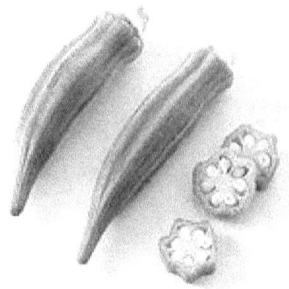

Okra vegetable

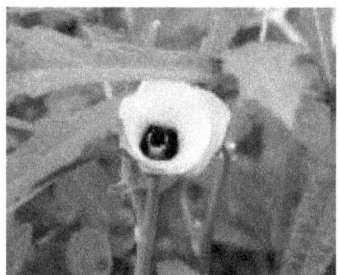

Okra plant

- Mike Warren from San Antonio, Texas, writes:

I have grown it several years, both in-ground in the traditional soil garden and several times in hydroponic planters. Both plantings always reach 6 or 7 feet in height with some plants topping out at 9 to 10 feet and still producing. In fact the only thing that I figure stopped it growing was the fact that I could no longer easily harvest the okra pods without damaging the plants, so the pods matured and the plant stopped growing and died.

Clemson Spineless is the variety of Okra I have growing in my "in ground" garden as well as in my "hydroponic" garden, both out doors and in my back yard. The hydroponic okra only reached a height (plant height) of a little over 8 feet, but the in ground okra is over 9 feet and still growing (now approaching 10 ft, Sep. 10). I pickle most of it with a simple recipe: [see recipe for "Pickled Okra" by M. Warren below in Recipes section].

Picking every other day or so, I am able to get over a case (12 pint jars) of pickled okra on a weekly basis, which I am told is much better than store bought pickled okra. This is the first year I have grown a garden in this soil, so it is virgin. It has been often over 100 F degrees so I water on a timer 15 to 30 minutes 6 AM and 6 PM with weekly feedings (in line to the sprinkler) of Miracle Grow or Peters water soluble fertilizer (Peters is preferred as it also has micro-nutrients and is less expensive). Also, my okra may be just a bit taller than others in my neighborhood but I have seen several gardens within a 10 block radius of my house with 8 foot to 9 foot tall okra plants (by appearance, not measurement).

- Jim Fruth from Pequot Lakes, Minnesota, writes:

When I farmed in the Central Valley foothills of California, ten foot tall (and multi-branched) okra was common. I planted in trenches down the mountain and irrigated with a hose running from the top of the hill to the bottom. Today, as a Northern Minnesota farmer, I sell okra at my produce stand whenever I can coax a crop out of it. Jim proves that okra lovers are found everywhere.

- Heather Tutorow from Modesto, California has this to say:
My grandparents moved to Modesto, CA in 1950. My grandpa as long as I can remember has had at least an acre of okra. Right after they moved to Modesto my grandfather woke up one morning to find several Sheriff's officers tromping through the okra and stepping on the watermelon. He went out to see what was up. The Sheriff was convinced that my grandpa was growing pot in his garden and had never heard of, let alone seen okra. It took a couple cups of coffee and a few of last years pickled okras to send this law officer on his way. He later became a close friend of the family. Much like everyone who has ever crossed paths with grandpa. It just isn't summer without okra.

For those who think they can do better than the Sheriff, see the picture below. Might you be confused, also?

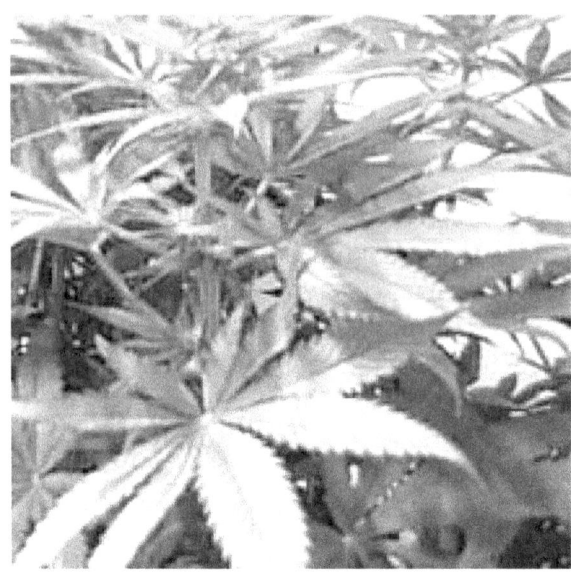

How to freeze Okra

Start with freshly picked okra. Wash, cut the stems off, being careful not to cut into seed chamber, otherwise the seeds may spill out. Blanch by putting into rapidly boiling water for about 3 minutes. Remove and cool immediately by placing under cool running water. Pat dry, optionally make a cut lengthwise, pack in plastic bags, seal tightly and place in the freezer. Should keep well up to a year.

An alternate method is suggested by Pam from Colorado: "I wash the okra and slice it into 1/4 -1/2" pieces, shake it in corn meal and freeze it in plastic bags in meal sized portions. I only ever fry it so that technique works great for me."
****

Okra Seed Sources

If you're starting out, please check at your local garden center or hardware store. They usually have at least a couple of varieties suited to your local conditions. An old standby is "Clemson Spineless", available throughout the U.S.

The following is a list of some places that sell okra seeds. These are mainly for your information only.

Park Seeds
Park Seed Company
1 Parkton Ave
Greenwood, SC 29647
eMail: info@parkscs.com
Ph: 800-213-0076

eSeeds.com
eSeeds.com Ltd
Blenheim House
2 Church Road
Milton under Wychwood, Oxfordshire
United Kingdom OX7 6LF
Tel: +44 (0)1993 830 399
Fax: +44 (0)1993 831 397

Ferry Morse Seeds
   **US company who sells through major stores like Lowe's
Toll free ph 1-800-283-3400**

Melissa's (CHINESE OKRA)
Corporate Office:
Melissa's/World Variety Produce, Inc.
P.O. Box 21127
Los Angeles, CA 90021
eMail: hotline@melissas.com
Phone: (800) 588-0151

Namdhari Seeds (INDIAN VARIETIES)
Uday Singh, Managing Director
EMAIL: UDAYSINGH@NAMDHARISEEDS.COM

Seed Savers (HEIRLOOM VARIETIES)

3094 North Winn Road
Decorah, IA 52101
Ph: 563-382-5990
Fax: 563-382-5872
eMail: tara@seedsavers.org

Tropilab (TROPICAL PLANT SEEDS)
    6428 18TH AVENUE NORTH
    St. Petersburg, FL 33710–5528, USA
    E mail: *info@tropilab.com*
    Phone: (727) 344 - 7608
    E-Fax: (708) 575 1761
    Toll free: (877)808-9410 (for ordering only)

APPENDIX A

QUIZ ON MYTH AND REALITY OF VEGETARIANISM

How much do you know about scientific validity of vegetarianism. Answer the following questions as myth (M) or reality (R) and compare your answers at the end. Take this quiz, then read the guide, if you have not already done so, to make yourself knowledgeable about nutrition in general, and vegetarianism in particular.

1. Vegetarians are not as healthy as non-vegetarians.

2. Vegetarians do not need dietary fiber.

3. Vegetarian foods cannot provide complete protein.

4. Balanced vegetarian foods can provide proteins as good as meat.

5. Vegetarians always suffer from stomach gas.

6. Vegetarian foods are difficult to digest and it takes a while for the digestive system to adjust to extra dietary fiber.

7. Vegetarian diets are more effective than non-vegetarian for losing or controlling weight.

8. Fruits, whole grains and raw vegetables take more chewing than meat and white bread.

9. More chewing makes you eat more.

10. People become vegetarians due to religious and humanitarian reasons only.

11. Over 75 % of deaths in the U.S. that occur from heart ailments, stroke, and cancer can be reduced by adopting a vegetarian diet.

12. Vegetarian diets have to be completely meat-free for providing beneficial effects.

13. Vegetarians can smoke without ill effects.

14. Green and yellow vegetables are helpful against cancer related to smoking.

15. By-pass surgery is the only way to save heart patients, and diet-exercise treatments are normally ineffective.

16. Vegetarian diets can lower cholesterol.

17. Excessive calories from fruits and vegetables are not fattening.

18. Once you learn to live normally with food containing good amounts of fruits, vegetables and whole grains, you don't have to exercise for the sake of maintaining a normal weight.

19. Fat children normally grow up to be fat adults, because they possess a higher number of fat cells.

20. The vitamins from fruits and vegetables are chemically better than synthetic vitamins.

21. Living exclusively on vegetables and fruits may cause deficiency of vitamin B 12 and D.

22. Including milk in your diet can supply vitamin B 12 and D.

23. Saturated fats and cholesterol that cause heart problems and cancer are provided mainly by meat.

24. Vegetarian foods are almost lacking in fat and cholesterol.

25. Fruits, vegetables and whole grains can reduce the chances of constipation and intestinal ailments.

26. People in developed countries eat healthier foods due to advancements in food processing and preservation.

27. Vegetarians cannot compete in sports with meat eaters.

28. Meat eaters live longer than vegetarians.

29. The biological and evolutionary evidence supports us as meat eaters.

30. Vegetarian foods provide an economical source of protein.

31. Our digestive tract is more suitable for plant foods.

32. Our teeth are more suitable for eating meat than tubers and seeds.

33. Many researchers in the West are ignorant about eating attitudes of earlier societies.

34. Protein in milk and eggs is used more efficiently than that in meat.

35. You cannot get fat by eating excessive protein.

36. Good consumption of vegetarian foods can meet calcium requirements.

37. Meat is required at every meal to meet protein requirements.

38. It is always good to take as many vitamins as possible.

39. It is hard to be a fat vegetarian.

40. Vegetarians are food faddists.

41. Vegetarian diets are low in saturated fat and calories.

42. Vegetarians eating fried vegetables can get fat.

43. Vegetarians can consume a lot of sugar in sweets or otherwise without getting fat.

44. High meat diets overdose on protein and ignore carbohydrates.

45. Fruits, vegetables and whole grains provide too much carbohydrates that fatten us.

46. You are too old to be a vegetarian now.

47. Fries are potatoes--a vegetable, so not fattening.

48. A large salad before dinner is a useful low-calorie method of filling yourself up.

49. Exercise increases your appetite.

50. Low-fat cooking methods (steaming, broiling etc.) can reduce calorie-intake.

ANSWERS: (1) M; (2) R; (3) M; (4) R; (5) M; (6) R; (7) R; (8) R; (9) M; (10)M; (11) R; (12) M; (13) M; (14) R; (15) M; (16) R; (17) M; (18) R; (19) R; (20) M; (21) R; (22) R; (23) R; (24) R; (25) R; (26) M; (27) M; (28) M; (29) M; (30) R; (31) R; (32) M; (33) R; (34) R; (35) M; (36) R; (37) M; (38) M; (39) R; (40) M; (41) R; (42) R; (43) M; (44) R; (45) M; (46) M; (47) M; (48) R; (49) M; (50) R.

APPENDIX B

EXAMPLES OF NUTRITIONALLY BALANCED VEGETARIAN MENUS

The menus 1 to 4 were devised by the New York City Department of Health's Bureau of Nutrition. Menus 1, 2 are for ovolacto- and 3, 4, for lactovegetarians. These are designed to provide adequate protein and the daily requirements of vitamins and minerals without overloading on saturated fats, cholesterol, and calories. The average calorie supply is about 2,400 daily. The menus 5 and 6 were devised by the Department of Nutrition of the School of Health at Loma Linda University, California. These provide 2,800 to 2,900 calories a day and about 80 grams of protein each. If you need to reduce calories, adjust by changing portion size or cut down on fats or follow menus 7 and 8 which provide 1200 and 1500 calories and 69 and 84 grams of protein, respectively. For recipes on the selected items in these menus and for other recipes on natural vegetarian diets see Dhillon, *Health Happiness and Longevity: Eastern and Western Approach,* Japan Publications, Tokyo/Harper & Row, New York, 1983.

SAMPLE MENU 1

BREAKFAST:
Cantaloupe 1/2 medium
Shredded-wheat biscuit 2
Whole-grain or enriched toast 1 slice
Margarine 1 pat (1 tsp)
Skim milk 1 cup

LUNCH:
Vegetable juice 1 cup
Egg-salad sandwich; 1

2 slices whole grain bread
1 medium egg
1 tablespoon diced celery
1 teaspoon mayonnaise
Pear 1 medium

SNACK:
Dried apricot halves 4
Almonds 1/4 cup

DINNER:
Soy and brown-rice loaf 1 cup
Carrots 1/2 cup
Broccoli 1/2 cup
Margarine 1 pat (1 tsp)
Waldorf salad: 6 oz.
1/2 cup diced apple
1 tablespoon diced celery
I tablespoon raisins
1 tablespoon chopped walnuts
1 tablespoon mayonnaise
Vanilla pudding 1/2 cup

SNACK:
Buttermilk or yogurt 1 cup
Graham crackers 4

SAMPLE MENU 2

BREAKFAST:
Grapefruit 1/2
Sliced cheese biscuit 1 oz.
Whole-grain or enriched toast 2 slices
Margarine 1 pat (1 tsp)
Skim milk 1/2 cup

LUNCH:
Black beans and rice 1 cup
Mixed green salad
Cottage cheese 1/2 cup
Salad dressing 1 tbsp
Whole grain or enriched bread 1 slice
Margarine 1 pat
Cantaloupe 1 slice

SNACK:
Yogurt 1 cup
Sunflower seeds 1/4 cup

DINNER:
Potato kugel 1 cup
Baked acorn squash 1/2 CUP
Coleslaw 1/2 cup
Mayonnaise 1 teaspoon
Whole-grain or enriched bread 1 slice
Margarine 1 pat
Pear 1 medium

SNACK:
Milk 1/2 cup
Bulger wheat 3/4 cup
Raisins 1/4 cup

SAMPLE MENU 3

BREAKFAST:
Grapefruit juice 1/2 cup
Oatmeal 1 cup
Whole-grain or enriched toast 1 slice
Margarine 1 teaspoon
Skim milk 1/2 cup

SNACK:
Yogurt 1/2 cup
Sesame bread sticks 4-6

LUNCH:
Grilled cheese sandwich: 1
2 slices whole-grain toast
1 ounce cheese
1 pat margarine
Tossed green salad
Salad dressing 1 tablespoon
Fresh fruit cup 1 cup

SNACK:
Raisins 1/4 cup
Peanuts 1/4 cup

DINNER:
Tomato juice 1/2 cup
Mixed bean salad 1 cup
Pancake delight
Apple 1 medium

SNACK:
Whole grain or enriched cereal 1 cup
Milk 1/2 cup

SAMPLE MENU 4

BREAKFAST:
Orange 1 medium
Cottage cheese 1/4 cup
Whole-grain or enriched toast 2 slices
Margarine 1 pat (1 tsp)
Skim milk 1/2 cup

SNACK:
Part-skimmed cheese 1 slice
Whole grain or enriched crackers 4-6

LUNCH:
Split-pea soup, 1 cup
Sesame crackers
Tomato and cucumber salad
Salad dressing 1 tbsp
Baked apple
Skim milk 1/2 cup

SNACK:
Prunes 2
Roasted soybeans 1/4 cup

DINNER:
Fresh fruit cup
Baked macaroni and cheese 1 cup
Collard greens 1/2 cup
Whole grain or enriched bread 1 slice
Margarine 2 pats
Junket 1/2 cup

SNACK:
Whole gram or enriched roll 1
Buttermilk 1/2 cup

SAMPLE MENU 5

BREAKFAST:
Orange 1 medium
Oatmeal (1/3 cup dry) with
1 tablespoon molasses
1/4 cup raisins
2/3 cup nondairy creamer or powdered soy milk

Whole-wheat toast 2 slices
Margarine 2 teaspoons
Peanut butter 1 tablespoon

LUNCH:
Savory patties 2 servings
Baked potato 1
Margarine 1 tablespoon
Cooked turnip greens 1 cup
Large tomato, sliced 1
Whole-wheat bread 1 slice
Margarine 1 teaspoon

DINNER:
Wheat tortillas with filling 2 servings
Apple 1 medium
Figs 5 large dried
Raw almonds 15

SAMPLE MENU 6

BREAKFAST:
Orange 1 medium
Whole-wheat cooked cereal,
1 cup with molasses
1/4 cup raisins
1/3 cup nondairy creamer or powdered soy milk
Banana 1
Whole-wheat toast 2 slices
Margarine 2 teaspoons
Peanut butter 2 tablespoons

LUNCH:
Black beans on rice 2 servings
Diced carrots, cooked 1/2 cup or Summer squash, diced 1 cup
Coleslaw 2/3 cup

Date bread 2 slices

DINNER:
Thick vegetable soup 2 servings
Kale (no stems) cooked 3/4 cup
Whole-wheat bread 1 slice
Margarine 1 teaspoon

SAMPLE MENU 7

BREAKFAST:
Orange juice 1/2 cup
Toast 1 slice
Margarine 1/2 teaspoon
Skim milk 1 cup

SNACK:
Skim milk 1/2 cup

LUNCH:
Pea soup 1 cup
Open broiled cheese sandwich 1 (2 oz skim cheese: Mozzarella, or sapsago)
Large cucumber, green pepper, as desired carrot, onion and tomato salad
Fresh pear 1 small
Skim milk 1 cup

SNACK:
Sliced banana 1/2 small
Iced or hot tea/lemon as desired

DINNER:
Broccoli or spinach quiche 1 slice
Fresh relish plate as desired
Apple 1 small

Non-fat milk 1 cup

SNACK:
Skim milk 1/2 cup

SAMPLE MENU 8

BREAKFAST:
Applesauce 1/2 cup
Toast 1 slice
Margarine 1/2 teaspoon
Skim milk 1 cup

SNACK:
Dried apricots 1/2 cup

LUNCH:
Low-fat yogurt 1/2 cup with herbs to make dressing for salad
Steamed mixed vegetables as desired with rice
Margarine 1/2 teaspoon
Large green salad with sprouts as desired
Fruit salad 1 cup
Skim milk 1 cup

SNACK:
Tangerine 1 large

DINNER:
Omelet with 1/3 cup low-fat 1 egg
cottage cheese
Bread 2 slices
Margarine 1 teaspoon
Black beans with large fresh 2/3 cup spinach salad with chopped
radishes and cucumbers
Fresh grapes 12
Skim milk 1 cup

SNACK:
Yogurt sprinkled with wheat germ 1/2 cup
Grapenuts (cereals) as desired

APPENDIX C

EXAMPLES OF VGETARIAN DIET RECIPES

The following pages include selective recipes, mostly of wholesome natural foods. The recipes are carefully balanced, with equal emphasis on healthful ingredients and appetizing flavors. There are too many recipes to list all of them. For more recipes on vegetarianism including additional recipes on Soups, Chutneys, Grains, Beverages, Fruits-Desserts, Italian and Indian gourmet recipes, and much more, please inquire about "Vegetarian Recipes" guide from dpcpress.com

VEGETARIAN MEALS
TOFU RECIPES
RECIPES FOR WESTERN STYLE FOODS
RAITA YOGURT
SALADS
DIPS AND DRESSINGS
SNACKS
****

VEGETARIAN MEALS

Vegetarian Chow Mein
1/2 pound dried or fresh egg noodles
2 ounces celery
2 ounces canned bamboo shoots
2 tablespoons peanut oil for Stir-frying
3 garlic cloves, crushed
1 small onion, finely sliced
1/2 pound small button mushrooms, whole
1 tablespoon light soy sauce
2 tablespoons dark soy sauce
2 teaspoons finely chopped fresh ginger
3 tablespoons vegetable stock

1 tablespoon rice wine or dry sherry
1 teaspoon sugar
1/4 pound bean sprouts
Garnish: Fresh coriander sprigs

If you are using fresh noodles, blanch them first in a large pot of boiling water for 3 to 5 minutes. If you are using the dried noodles, cook in boiling water for 4 to 5 minutes.
Drain the noodles, then put them into cold water until required.

String the celery and slice diagonally. Shred the bamboo shoots. Heat a wok or large frying-pan and add the oil. When moderately hot, add the garlic and stir-fry for 10 seconds. Add the onion, mushrooms, celery, and bamboo shoots and stir-fry for about 5 minutes.

Drain the noodles thoroughly and put into the wok. Continue to stir-fry for 1 minute then add the rest of the ingredients except the bean sprouts. Continue to stir-fry for another 2 minutes and then add the bean sprouts. Give the mixture a good stir and turn it onto a serving platter.
Garnish with fresh coriander sprigs.
Serves 4
Per Serving is about 335 Calories and only 15% from Fat.

Vegetarian Enchilada Casserole
28 ounces canned crushed tomatoes in tomato puree
14 1/2 ounces canned chunky salsa
6 ounces canned tomato paste
30 ounces canned black beans, rinsed and drained
15 1/4 ounces canned whole kernel corn, drained
4 ounces canned diced green chilies
1 1/2 tablespoons ground cumin
1/2 teaspoon garlic powder 5 corn tortillas
2 1/4 ounces canned sliced ripe olives, drained

1. In a large bowl, combine the tomatoes, salsa, tomato paste, beans, corn, green chilies, cumin, and garlic powder. Mix well. Ladle about 1 cup of this mixture in to the bottom of a 4-quart electric slow cooker; spread evenly. Top with 1 1/4 tortillas, cutting to fit as necessary. Spread on 1/4 of the remaining tomato mixture. Repeat these layers 2 more times, ending with the rest of the tomato mixture; spread evenly over the top. Sprinkle the sliced olives over all.
2. Cover and cook on the low heat setting about 5 hours.
Serve hot. Serves 5 to 6

Layered Dinner
6 potatoes, sliced
1 large onion, sliced
2 carrots, sliced
1 green pepper, sliced
1 zucchini, sliced
1 cup corn, frozen or fresh
1 cup peas, frozen or fresh Optional Vegetables mushrooms broccoli green beans Sauce
2 1/2 cups tomato sauce
1/4 cup tamari, low-sodium
1 teaspoon thyme, ground
1 teaspoon dry mustard
1 teaspoon basil
2 teaspoons chili powder
1/2 teaspoon cinnamon
1/8 teaspoon sage
2 tablespoons parsley flakes

Layer vegetables in large casserole in order given. Mix together ingredients for sauce and pour over vegetables. Cook 6 hours at high or 12 at low.

Vegetarian Stew
1/2 cup mushrooms
1 tablespoon vegetable oil
1/2 cup canned bamboo shoots, sliced and drained
1 8 oz can sliced water chestnuts, drained
1 carrot, julienned (cut in long thin strips)
3 cups shredded Napa cabbage
3 cups Vegetable Broth
2 ounces bean threads, or mung vermicelli
1 cup firm tofu, cut in 1/2-inch cubes
16 snow peas, strings removed, julienned
2 cups fresh bean sprouts
3 tablespoons soy sauce
2 tablespoons cornstarch, mixed well with
4-5 Tbls cold water
1 teaspoon Oriental sesame oil
2 to 3 cups hot water

In a wok, stir-fry mushrooms, bamboo shoots, water chestnuts, carrot, and cabbage, in oil on high for 4 minutes. Add broth, and bean threads. Reduce heat, cover, and simmer for 5 minutes.

Add tofu, snow peas, bean sprouts, and soy sauce. Cover and simmer for 2 minutes. Stir in cornstarch mixture and continue to cook until sauce thickens. Drizzle with sesame oil and serve.

Serves 6
Per Serving is about 238 Calories - Calories From: Fat 27%, Protein 18%, Carbohydrate 55%

Paneer peas pilau
It's a gourmet meal of India. It is pretty much balanced meal. Protein from the peas and paneer (kind of cheese), carbohydrate from the rice and some, but not too much, fat - most of it unsaturated. Pilau makes a nice meal on it's own but you might find it a little dry, in

which case I would suggest a raita (yogurt-based dish) and or some dhal to go with it. Of course you can serve it with anything you like.

1 mug of long-grain rice
1.6 mugs of water A large handful of green peas (fresh or frozen)
50 - 70g of paneer
Half a teaspoon of ground coriander
Salt
Oil

Put the rice, peas, salt and water into a pan and stir gently to separate the rice grains. Bring to the boil then turn down the heat to minimum. Give the rice another gentle stir and put a lid on the pan tightly. It should take twenty minutes or so for the rice to cook and absorb all the water. Try not to disturb it during this time. If you want to try it to see if it's cooked, lift a few grains out with a fork.

When the rice is ready, turn off the heat and leave the pan covered while you prepare the paneer. Cut the paneer into 1 cm cubes and fry it in oil with the coriander until it is beginning to go golden. About five minutes on a medium heat should do it. Stir the paneer and the oil into the rice and peas mixture. Your pilau is now ready to serve.

Try replacing paneer with tofu cubes with equally good results.

Vegetable Lasagna
6 lasagna noodles
1 cup ricotta cheese
1 cup cottage cheese, drained
2 eggs
1/2 cup Parmesan cheese
1/2 teaspoon salt
1/4 teaspoon pepper
1 cup chopped red pepper
1 cup chopped green pepper
1 chopped onion

2 cloves garlic, minced
2 tablespoons olive oil
1 carrot, grated
1 zucchini, grated
1 16 oz. can whole tomatoes
1 6 oz. can tomato paste
1/3 cup red wine
2 teaspoons parsley flakes
2 teaspoons salt
2 teaspoons sugar
1 teaspoon basil
1 teaspoon oregano
2 bay leaves
3 cups grated mozzarella cheese

Cook the lasagna noodles according to the package directions. Then put the noodles in cold water and set them aside.

In a bowl that doesn't have to be microwave-safe, combine the ricotta cheese, cottage cheese, eggs, Parmesan cheese, salt, and pepper. Stir until the ingredients are mixed and set the bowl aside.

Then in a microwave-safe bowl combine the peppers, onion, garlic, and oil. Microwave the vegetables for 5 to 6 minutes, until the vegetables are tender. Stir the carrot and zucchini into the cooled vegetables. Set the bowl aside for a bit.

Smash the tomatoes a little with a fork. Then stir in the tomato paste and the wine, until the mixture is pretty smooth. You can substitute water or grape juice for the wine or any other liquid. Mix in the parsley, salt, sugar, basil, oregano, and bay leaves. Microwave the mixture on high for 10 minutes. Fish out the bay leaves and discard them.

Grease a 9x13 pan. Cover the bottom of the dish with noodles and make layers of ricotta, vegetables, mozzarella, and sauce. End with a layer of mozzarella cheese on top and spoon some tomato sauce over the cheese. Microwave for 5 minutes, then let them stand for 10

minutes to set before eating.
Serves 8
You can make the lasagna rolls, if you don't mind extra work and time.

Brown Basmati Rice
1 cup brown basmati rice
1 cup water
1\2 cup white wine
1\4 cup frozen peas 1 clove garlic (chopped) 1 t fresh ginger (chopped) 1 t olive oil 1 T chopped parsley optional: 1 t curry powder. Wash and rinse rice and set aside. Sauté ginger and garlic with oil and 1 t of water in saucepan for 1 minute. Add rice and stir while sautéing for 30 sec over high heat. Add water and curry powder and boil moderately until rice begins to pit. Add wine and frozen peas and keep heat up just until it comes back to a boil. Cover tightly and turn the heat down to simmer and let cook for 20 minutes. Turn off heat and leave pot covered on burner for another 15 minutes. Serve and sprinkle parsley over top. Goes well with the curried beans and other vegetables; the recipes for some are given below.

Curried Beans
1 green bell pepper, chopped 1 cup black beans, cooked 3 roma tomatoes, diced 1\2 cup frozen corn 1 cup canned or fresh pineapple chunks 1/2 t ginger, chopped 1 t curry powder pinch of cinnamon pinch of nutmeg Heat it all up in a saucepan, thinning it with any left over pineapple juice or water. Serve over brown basmati rice.

Curried Garbanzos
1 cup cooked garbanzo beans (chickpeas) 2 large carrots, chopped 1 stalk celery, chopped 1 small parsnip, chopped. 1 large potato, diced

into 1\2 in. cubes 1 can stewed tomatoes. 1 packet vegetable bouillon. 4 scallions, chopped 1 T curry powder 1/4 t nutmeg pinch of cinnamon pinch of cayenne (optional) Cook in large saucepan for 30 min. Add a little water if needed. Serve over brown basmati rice, to give the balanced protein (legume and grain). Goes well with mixed vegetable salad.

Pea Soup
3 cups water 2 T dried yellow peas 1 t pot barley 1 yellow onion, chopped coarsely 1 carrot (sliced thinly) 1 stalk of celery (minced) 1 clove garlic chopped vegetables (broccoli stalks or whatever is available) 1 stick of astragalus 1 bay leaf 1\4 t cayenne pepper several parsley stalks (chopped fine) soy, tamari, miso or Ketjap manis to taste Sauté onion till browned and add astragalus, cayenne, bay leaf, peas, barley, parsley stalks and water and simmer for at least 2 hours with lid on. Add carrot, celery and vegetables and simmer for 1 more hour. When ready to serve, remove astragalus and bay leaf and add soy sauce to serving bowl (not to pot)

Red Curry Beans
1 diced onion
3 cloves garlic
1/4 t nutmeg 1\4 t cinnamon 1/2 t cloves cayenne pepper to taste 1 cup cooked kidney beans 4 roma tomatoes (chopped) 1 cup short grained rice 3\4 cup water 1\2 cup white wine Sauté onion and garlic in a frying pan in a little olive oil until onions are clear and add spices. Put beans in pan, sauté around a little bit, add tomatoes, rice and water. Simmer until water is absorbed then add wine, cover and simmer 30 min.

Vegan Chili
1 large jalapeno pepper, diced finely

2 bell peppers, (one green and one red/yellow)
1 cup kidney beans
1 chopped onion
2 garlic cloves
3 chopped roma tomatoes
cumin, coriander, oregano to taste
1 T olive oil Soak the beans overnight, then simmer until tender (1 to 2 hours). Chop onions and garlic, sauté in oil. Add peppers, sauté with onion and garlic. Add chopped tomatoes, cook until soft. Add the beans, and some bean liquid. Add the spices and cook for another hour or so.

Vegetable Curry
1 large onion, chopped
2 shiitake mushrooms, sliced
1 T. curry powder

1/4 t ginger 1 large carrot, sliced 1 stalk celery, sliced 1 cup green beans, sliced 1 bell pepper, chopped 1 cup cauliflower, in bite-sized pieces 1 cup broccoli, in bite-sized pieces 1 small butternut squash, diced into 1\2 in. cubes 2 T raisins 1 small parsnip, chopped 1\ 2 cup water. Brown onion in skillet , stir in curry, ginger, mushrooms and water and cook until liquid is reduced to a sauce. Let sit on warm burner while you steam the rest of the ingredients until they are hot but still have a raw crunchy texture (about 10 min). Serve veggies over rice and pour the curry sauce over the vegetables. Serves 6
****

TOFU RECIPES

Tofu Walnut Cutlets At it's simplest, it's just finely chopped raw onion and walnuts mashed into tofu and fried as cutlets. It's very tasty like that, so if you haven't the time don't bother with the detailed recipe below. These cutlets are high in protein and extremely low in fat (they don't absorb much oil in frying either).

Unlike other pulses, soy beans contain most of amino acids needed by the body to synthesize proteins and the addition of oats, nuts and seeds makes very nutritious cutlets indeed. They can be frozen to fry them later. Lay them on baking paper on a tray and put into the freezer. Don't lay them too close side by side or they'll stick together, but you can layer them with sheets of paper in between. Once they have frozen, put the cutlets into plastic bags, with the bags closed, leave in the freezer until required. They keep for 4 or 5 weeks. 1 kg tofu 200g shelled walnuts 1 large onion 3 cloves of garlic 1 mug of porridge oats 1 dessert spoon of soy sauce 3 teaspoons mixed seeds e.g. Poppy seed, sesame, coriander, mustard 1 teaspoon of salt Vegetable oil for frying Peel and finely chop the onion and garlic (keep them separate). Chop the walnuts finely too. Heat a very little vegetable oil in a frying pan until it is really hot. Watch for it beginning to smoke - that's it ready. Take the pan off the heat and throw in the seeds. They should start to pop. Add the onions immediately and stir - the pan will still be very hot so stir the onions around for a few minutes while it cools a little - you don't want to burn the seeds. Return the pan to the flame (turn the heat down a bit) and continue stirring. Add the walnuts, oats and garlic once the onions are transparent, and continue stirring for about 5-7 minutes. Turn off the heat and let the pan stand while you prepare the tofu.

Rinse the tofu in cold water, put it in a pot or large bowl (something with a flat bottom is best) and mash it with a potato masher or something similar. Add the salt, soy sauce (and some red or black pepper if you like) and the contents of the frying pan. Mash it all together well. Make burger or sausage shapes with the mix and fry until golden brown (about 4 minutes either side).

Braised Tofu 1\2 pound firm tofu, cut into 1\2 in. cubes 1 cup chopped vegetables (broccoli, cauliflower, shallots, carrots etc) 1\2 t olive oil sauce 1\4 cup tamari sauce (or substitute 3 T Ketjap manis) 1\2 t balsamic vinegar 1 t finely chopped ginger 3 cloves crushed garlic Marinate tofu in sauce mixture for one hour or more. Braise tofu by adding some sauce mixture in frying pan with olive oil. Turn gently and reduce.

Tofu Strips

1 block soft tofu 1 T tamari sauce 1/4 cup water Cut tofu into 1/4 thick slabs. Lay flat on dish and pour soy sauce and water over it. Allow to marinate several hours or overnight, turning occasionally. 2 T engevita yeast 1 t parsley 2 cloves diced garlic 2 T finely chopped onion 2 T whole wheat flour cayenne pepper to taste Mix dry ingredients together and place on a shallow plate.

Coat the marinated tofu strips in the mixture. Wipe a cookie sheet with olive oil and place the coated cubes on the tray. Bake in a 400F oven for 45 minutes, or until lightly browned.

Tofu with Wine

1/2 pound extra firm tofu. 1\4 cup wheat flour 1 T olive oil 1/2 cup white wine 1 small onion ,chopped 1 cup broccoli florets, chopped 1 clove garlic, minced 1\4 t cayenne 1 cup soymilk 1 T cornstarch Slice tofu into 1\4 in strips Roll the tofu in the flour till coated. Heat the oil in a large saucepan, and put the strips in. Cook over moderate heat until strips are browned on underside, then turn and brown on the other side. Remove from saucepan and set aside. Add the wine, broccoli, onion and garlic to the saucepan. Sauté until onion is just soft, a minute or two. Mix the cornstarch with the soymilk and wine. Add the tofu strips back to the pan, then add the soymilk mixture. Stir until soymilk thickens. Add more soymilk if it is too dry. Reduce the heat and simmer about a minute. Serve over rice or potatoes.
****

RECIPES FOR WESTERN STYLE FOODS

Bean Burgers You can make these in quantity and freeze them for future use. Soybeans or any kind of beans plus oatmeal can be used as the base of bean burgers. 1 cup raw beans 1 cup uncooked oatmeal 1/2 cup nutritional yeast 1/2 teaspoon garlic powder 1 teaspoon dry mustard 1 teaspoon chili powder 1 teaspoon onion powder 2 tablespoons vegetable oil Cook beans, mash, and combine with oatmeal, yeast, garlic, mustard chili, and onion powder. Heat in oven for a few minutes at 300° F. (150° C.). (This inhibits soaking up oil during sautéing.) Form into six thin burgers and fry in oil over low heat. Top with sliced onion and catsup and serve on bread or bun. Serves 6

Black Bean Burritos 1 cup cooked black beans 1 red bell pepper (chopped) 1 green bell pepper (chopped) 2 garlic cloves (chopped) tortillas Salsa Dip(Ready made or from recipe below) Combine beans, peppers, garlic and salsa Put into a tortilla and microwave until done **Salsa Dip** 5 roma tomatoes (chopped) 1 jalapeno pepper, (chopped) 1 bell pepper, (chopped), any color that you prefer-- yellow/red/green. 2 T finely chopped fresh cilantro

2 T finely chopped parsley 1 small red onion, (finely chopped) 2 cloves garlic, (minced) 1 t balsamic vinegar, (or lemon juice) Mix, chill and serve.

Black Bean Burgers
3 16-oz cans black beans, rinsed and drained 1 1/2 cups uncooked regular oats 1 medium onion, chopped 2 jalapeno peppers, seeded & chopped 3/4 cup chopped fresh cilantro 2 large eggs (or substitute), lightly beaten 1 teaspoon salt 1/4 cup flour 1/4 cup cornmeal 1 tablespoon vegetable oil 8 hamburger buns condiments of choice Coarsely mash beans with a fork. Combine beans and other ingredients; shape into 8 patties. Stir together flour and cornmeal and dredge patties in mixture. Cook patties in hot oil in a large non-stick skillet over medium-high heat for 5 minutes on each side or until

lightly browned. Drain on paper towels. Serve on buns with condiments of choice (lettuce, tomato, onion, mayo, ketchup, mustard, salsa, etc.).

****

RAITA YOGURT

This is an Indian side dish - good for serving with spicy food, but equally good on its own as a refreshing snack. The ingredients can vary. The yogurt-based sauce is the defining characteristic and makes this dish excellent for the digestive system. We suggest non-fat yogurt for weight watchers. Here are some of favorite raita recipes. Feel free to experiment with your own combinations. You won't go far wrong. **Mixed raita** 1 small cucumber, peeled 2 tomatoes 1/2 an onion 1/2 tsp. each of whole cumin seed and whole mustard seed, roasted and pounded 1/4 tsp. red chilli powder A pinch of salt 250-300g of natural yogurt Chop the vegetables finely and mix everything together. That's it.

Potato raita
2 medium potatoes 1/2 an onion 1/2 tsp. whole mustard seeds, roasted and pounded 1 sprig or 5 or 6 leaves of fresh mint A pinch of salt 250g natural yogurt (non-fat for weight watchers) Boil the whole potatoes with skin or use microwave. You can stick a fork in them to check if done. Leave these to cool down. Chop the onion and mint finely and mix everything together except the potatoes which will still be cooling. After a few minutes, drain the potatoes, cut into 1 cm cubes, rinse in cold water and add to the mixture. It doesn't matter if they are still a little warm.

Onion raita
Half an onion

A quarter tsp. each of black mustard seeds and cumin seeds A good pinch of dried mint Salt 200g of yogurt Grate the onion (use the side with the smallest holes if you're using that kind of grater), roast and pound the seeds and mix everything together. Tomato and coriander raita 4 firm tomatoes A small bunch of green coriander Half of a small onion A pinch each of red chilli and dried mint Salt 250-300g of yogurt Chop the tomatoes quite finely and pour off any excess juice and seeds. Grate, or finely chop, the onion and chop the coriander. Mix everything together.
****

SALADS

Arabic Salad 2 diced roma tomatoes 1 zucchini, peeled and chopped 1/2 onion chopped very fine 2 t cumin cilantro and cayenne to taste 2 T lemon juice 1 T olive oil 1 t flax oil drops sesame oil Toss and refrigerate. Serve with parsley sprigs. For easy digestion: Steam chopped onion, zucchini and tomato for 6 minutes. Chill and mix with other ingredients.

Cooked Carrot and Asparagus Salad
2 med. carrots 1\2 lb asparagus 1 T olive oil 1 t flax oil 1 small red onion thinly sliced pinch of cayenne pepper pinch of caraway seed sprigs of cilantro and parsley juice from one lemon. Cut carrots in 2-inch sticks 1\4 in. thick. Simmer carrots in olive oil and a bit of water over medium heat until tender. Remove and add asparagus to cooking liquid and simmer for 4 minutes. Remove asparagus. Reserve cooking liquid and rinse asparagus with cold water. Sauté onions in olive oil for 10 minutes. Add 1/2 cup vegetable cooking liquid, pepper and caraway seeds, and carrots and simmer for 5 minutes. Mix in asparagus. Add lemon juice, flax oil, parsley and cilantro just before serving. Can be served hot or cold.

88
Tofu Salad

this is to replace egg salad for sandwiches 1 block firm tofu 4 T prepared mustard 1 stalk celery 1 red bell pepper 1/4 t curry powder add cilantro to taste Chop tofu into small cubes. Chop pepper and celery into similar size as tofu. Mix everything and refrigerate.

Vegan Caesar salad
4 cloves garlic, to taste, chopped 1 lemon 1 T capers 4 T chickpeas (steamed) 1 t dry mustard 1 T tamari sauce 1 T olive oil 1 t flax oil croutons (optional) romaine lettuce Toss and serve with a few sprigs of parsley.

Coleslaw
1 small head finely sliced cabbage 1 stalk celery 1 red pepper 1 small carrot 1 scallion sprigs of parsley julienne pepper and carrot Finely chop celery, scallion and parsley 1 T balsamic vinegar juice from 1 lime 1 t dry mustard 1 t Ketjap manis (tamari or soy will do) 1 T pure maple syrup

dusting of cayenne 1/2 t caraway seed Toss and refrigerate

Cucumber Salad
2 med cucumbers 1 red onion 1 chopped roma tomato 1 t flax oil 1 T olive oil 2 T fresh basil 1 clove garlic (minced) 1 T balsamic vinegar several sprigs parsley Thin-slice the cucumbers and onion and put them in a container. Chop the basil and toss it in. Mix oil, garlic and vinegar and toss with the above ingredients. Refrigerate and add tomatoes and parsley when served.

Black Bean & Corn Salad
1\2 cup black beans, cooked 1 cup frozen corn. 1 medium onion. 1

red bell pepper. 5 cloves garlic. 1/4 cup fresh cilantro (chopped) 1 T olive oil. 1 t water. juice of one lemon, one lime, one orange Sauté pepper , garlic and onion for 3 minutes in olive oil and water. Mix other ingredients and sauté 1 minute with lid on. Pour into bowl and refrigerate for one hour. For easy digestion: Steam corn for 6 minutes first and cool.
****

DIPS AND DRESSINGS

Artichoke Dip 1 can artichoke hearts, diced 1\2 block extra firm tofu juice of one lime 2 garlic cloves, minced parsley, sage, rosemary and thyme to taste 2 T engevita yeast Blend every thing but the chokes in food processor or blender, adding just enough artichoke water to blend smoothly. Sprinkle extra nutritional yeast over the top, and bake at 250F for about an hour or until it cracks on top.

Bean Dip 1 cup pinto beans 2 chopped roma tomatoes 1 clove garlic, finely chopped 2 scallions, finely chopped 1 finely chopped jalapeno pepper pinch of cumin dash of lemon juice or balsamic vinegar Cook the beans to mush without burning them. Mix in other ingredients and chill. A double boiler or pressure cooker would do but beans will stick unless placed in a heat proof dish inside the cooker and covered with water. Set the dish on top of the trivet inside the cooker and put water below the trivet as well as in the dish.

Broccoli Dip 1 cup cooked broccoli stems (peeled) 1 T fresh-squeezed lemon juice 1/4 t curry powder 2 cloves garlic, minced 1 roma tomato, diced 1 scallion, sliced 1 jalapeno pepper, chopped In a food processor, blend the broccoli stems with the lemon juice, curry, garlic and pepper until completely smooth. Mix with the remaining ingredients and chill before serving.

Spicy Bean Dip

1\2 cup pinto beans 1\2 cup kidney beans 1 small can tomato paste 1 small onion 3 cloves garlic basil parsley apple juice or apple/lime juice to texture 1\2 t cayenne pepper Bring beans to a boil in a saucepan, boil for 5 minutes then pour off the water. Use fresh water and simmer until done. Drain beans and set aside This decreases the 'flatulent' effect of the beans. Sauté onion and garlic in the bottom of the pot with a little bit of olive oil for one minute. Put all ingredients into a food processor and blend coarsely.

Vegetarian Dip

1 large red onion 1/2 stalk of celery 1 green pepper 1 medium sized zucchini 1/4 teaspoon cayenne pepper 3 cloves of garlic 1/4 teaspoon chili powder 1/4 teaspoon cumin
1 T tahini paste
cilantro to taste juice of one lemon Chop onion, celery, tomatoes, green pepper and zucchini and put them in a cooking pan. Add cayenne, garlic, chili powder and cumin. Cook until vegetables are soft. Let them cool. Put them in the food processor with the remaining ingredients and mix.

Cucumber-tofu Dressing

1 cup soft tofu 2 T. capers juice of 1 lemon and 1 lime 1 long English cucumber 1 T finely chopped rosemary (works with dill or mint or a combination) whirl in blender until smooth.

Ginger Sauce 2 T fresh chopped ginger root. 1 T dry mustard. 1 T balsamic vinegar. 2 t Ketjap manis. 1 T Saki (white wine or sherry

will do fine) 1 t sesame oil 1 T olive oil 1 t flax oil cayenne pepper to taste Blend in blender or processor
****

SNACKS

Soy Nuts the perfect snack food Soak Soy beans overnight Lay flat on a baking tray or cookie sheet Roast in 350 degree F oven for 30 minutes or until the beans are browned to your taste. That's it. Use these nuts to replace popcorn, peanuts, crackerjacks or other snack foods.

Words of Wisdom

- "In a vegetarian world no one needs to worry about Kosher, Halal, Bird Flu, Mad Cow Disease and pollution from the waste of billions day to day killings."
- "What you eat in private; you will wear in public. If you must Binge, Binge on Vegetables."
- "Eat food. Not too much. Mostly Plants." It's that simple!
- "The food you eat can be either the safe & most powerful form of medicine or the slowest form of poison." Need to hang this up in my kitchen!
- "The doctor of the future will no longer treat the human frame with drugs, but rather will cure and prevent disease with Nutrition. Special exercises, breathing tips... included." True
- "There is no diet that will do what eating healthy does." DIET is a wrooong word!"
- "At the end of the day, your HEALTH is your RESPONSIBILITY." Health
- "Eat better, Feel better" –A Simple solution to Weight Problem
- "It's all about creating HEALTHY habits, rather than restrictions." Healthy
- "You are not HUNGRY you are BORED drink some water & LEARN the difference."
- "It's not about finding the right diet; it's about adopting the right lifestyle." Just live the healthy lifestyle.
- "It isn't a DIET; It is a LIFESTYLE." I keep telling people this...they have yet to believe me
- "MYTH: If you exercise, it doesn't matter what you eat! FACT: If you exercise, it matters even more what you eat!
- "I don't have an ultimate goal weight; because the scale does not define me. I define myself: ACTIVE, HEALTHY, HAPPY." :)
- "Take care of your body; it's the only place you have to live. And you should eat to live, not live to eat." ~Good reminder~
- "Love your body because...you cannot look after something that you hate." very true words
- "To Lose the Weight, You Gotta Change How You relate to Food." Psychology Today
- "If you eat what you've always eaten, you will weigh what you always weighted." Very true.
- "I am not fat. I'm just easy to see." ..lol
- "Food has replaced sex in my life. Now I can't even get into my own pants"...lol
- "The hardest life of all is your ASS from the couch.".. That's what I'm talking 'bout!!!..lol

- "I never dance naked because my body has parts that don't stop moving when the music does"..Wiggle wiggle wiggle..lol
- Dear extra fat in my body, you have 2 options: Make your way to my boobs, or gtof...lol...haha haha..haa
- "If we're not meant to have midnight snacks, why is there a light in the fridge." Yeah.....why is that? hehe.
- "The best six doctors anywhere and no one can deny it are sunshine, water, rest, air, exercise and DIET." Wonderful advice. Manage stress followed by diet and exercise...simple but??
- Eat Healthy: morning eat within 30 minutes of waking to jump-start metabolism - few bites of oatmeal or half banana afternoon-Eat light snack before your workout. Small bowl of oatmeal-banana- apple slices with peanut butter. After workout-Eat within 30 minutes so your body doesn't start burning muscle - protein- handful almonds or protein shake.

About the Author: Dr. Sukhraj S. Dhillon has an advanced degree in life sciences and molecular biology from the west and a fascination with yoga, breathing, religion and spirituality from the east crafted out of studies at Yale University, U.S.A. and Punjab University, India. He is one of the first authors who is uniquely qualified to present Eastern and Western synthesis of health issues. He has published over 12 books and 40 research papers, and has expressed his views in the news media and workshops. He has been the President, Chairman of the board, and life-trustee of a non-profit religious organization and has expressed his views in the congregation and at international seminars.